BIRTH
SHOCK

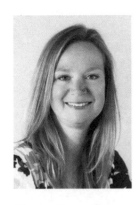

About the author

Mia Scotland is a Perinatal Clinical Psychologist and birth doula, working in private practice in the East Midlands, UK.

She has been helping mothers deal with birth trauma, perinatal depression and anxiety for more than 20 years. Her particular passion is for the psychology of birth and motherhood, from a biopsychosocial perspective. As well as running her private practice, she teaches birth professionals about the psychology of birth internationally. She has three children, and lives in Melton Mowbray, UK.

She is the author of *Why Postnatal Depression Matters*.

BIRTH SHOCK

HOW TO RECOVER FROM BIRTH TRAUMA
– WHY 'AT LEAST YOU'VE GOT A HEALTHY
BABY' ISN'T ENOUGH

MIA SCOTLAND

pinter
&
martin

Birth Shock: How to recover from birth trauma – why 'at least you've got a healthy baby' isn't enough

First published in the UK by Pinter & Martin Ltd 2020

Copyright © Mia Scotland 2020

ISBN 978-1-78066-495-8

Also available as an ebook

The right of Mia Scotland to be identified as the author of this work has been asserted by her in accordance with the Copyright, Designs and Patent Act of 1988

Edited by Susan Last
Index by Helen Bilton

British Library Cataloguing-in-Publication Data

A catalogue record for this book is available from the British Library

Printed in the EU by Hussar

This book has been printed on paper that is sourced and harvested from sustainable forests and is FSC accredited

Pinter & Martin Ltd
6 Effra Parade
London SW2 1PS

pinterandmartin.com

CONTENTS

PREFACE

At least you have a healthy baby. That, after all, is the most important thing. Or is it?

So why are you struggling to move on? Why does it matter to you? Why do you keep thinking about the birth, when you want to just move on and be a mother? And why do you feel guilty when other people say 'at least you have a healthy baby'?

If you're not sure of the answers, and you feel bad because you can't move on from the birth, then this book is for you.

Let me start by telling you a story. Last week, a friend of mine was walking home from work. He was approached by two other men, who harassed him and began to push him around, quite forcefully, trying to get a phone or money off him. They proceeded to hit and punch him. Someone intervened, and my friend managed to get away. He came home shaken and bruised.

When talking about it to others, he said 'I don't know why I'm still upset', and 'I should have been able to stop them. I feel so useless and weak'.

For the next part of the story, I want you to help me out. I'd like you to choose which of these two responses is most appropriate for this guy, in order to help him to get over his upset.

A 'Well, at least you've still got your phone and money.'

B 'Of course you're still upset. I would be if that had happened to me. And it wasn't your fault.'

It might be obvious to you why my friend was upset about being mugged, but not so obvious why you are upset about your birth. In this book, I aim to help you to understand why you are still upset about your birth. I also aim to help you to know and believe that it was not your fault. Finally, I would like you to feel and believe that you deserve massive respect for what you have coped with. This is what I do in my job as a perinatal clinical psychologist day in, day out. I help people recover from difficult births. I help people to believe that a healthy baby is not *all* that matters. You matter too.

TRIGGER WARNING: PLEASE TAKE CARE OF YOURSELF

This book is about birth trauma. If you have been traumatised, this means that reading this book might bring some of those memories to the fore for you. There are descriptions of traumatic births, with some graphic wording. There is also some discussion about sexual violence. This is especially true for Chapter 1.

If you feel that you want to avoid that chapter, please do. I think it's great that you are reading this book, and I really hope it helps. If there are times when you feel triggered, please take care of yourself. In Chapter 4 there are some 'grounding techniques' you can use. If the memory is still quite raw for you, I suggest that you read that chapter first, and remind yourself of, or equip yourself with, some techniques for taking care of your emotions while you read the book.

BIRTH IS A FEMINIST ISSUE

Birth is a feminist issue. What I mean by that, is that birth is about women. It is about women's rights, women's bodies, women's health, institutional power over women and their bodies, physical abuse of women, emotional abuse of women, sexual abuse of women, silencing of women, control of women, emancipation of women, empowerment of women, dignity of women, respect of women, and more. It is increasingly also about partners. Fathers are known to suffer trauma after witnessing their partners' births. It is also about babies, and about the best start for families. Most births happen in a hospital, within a health institution, with birth professionals attending. If you think birth trauma is just about birth, think again.

My clinical work, and research, suggests that birth trauma is a function of the systems that we birth in. These systems are arguably patriarchal, controlling, over-medicalised, and can be damaging to women's health, both physically and emotionally. I know that doctors and medicine do save lives. I'm not disputing the good that they do. But I am interested in the harm that they do, and that includes adding to the prevalence of birth trauma. That is why birth is a feminist issue.

To heal birth trauma, we need to take a close look at the system that birth trauma happens within. By helping you to see how the system made it worse for you, I will help you let go of some of the guilt or self-blame or confusion that you might be feeling right now, about your birth. It was not your fault. You did nothing wrong. Read on to see why I can emphatically say that to you, even though I don't even know you.

– 1 –

BIRTH AS WE KNOW IT IN OUR INDUSTRIALISED SOCIETY

THE ROLE OF PSYCHOLOGY: UNDERSTANDING OUR EVOLVED STRENGTHS

Human birth is something that we know very little about. That might seem an odd thing to say, but it's true. It has become such a hotbed of disputes, arguments and bizarre behaviour that we have got ourselves into quite a muddle when it comes to understanding how women and babies birth best. There are 'camps' that argue that birth as we know it should be eradicated, because it's such a painful ordeal and no modern or compassionate society should be putting women through that. There are 'camps' who argue that birth is a normal and joyous event that empowers women, and that modern medicine is crippling women by stealing that birthright from them through fear and obstetric intervention. Some believe that women birth in the same way as other mammals, and that they should be left in peace to do so. Others believe that all women need support through labour and that to leave her to it would be cruel. Some believe that women aren't evolved to birth well, because of the shape of our pelvis and the size of human heads, and so obstetric intervention is necessary. Some believe that the father needs to be there, while others believe that the father should not be there. And it goes on.

One thing that I have learned as a psychologist is that human beings are incredibly resourceful. Some species are less able to adapt to different environments, but humans can survive very toxic and challenging environments. There are three basic principles that I want to outline, when talking about birth. Firstly, there are many ways to give birth, and for that reason, different cultures do things differently. Secondly, cultural practices can be toxic to health. Some cultures do things that really are dangerous, and that includes during the perinatal period. Thirdly, some things are universally good for all humans, no matter what culture they are a part of. To help us to birth better, I think it's worth looking at these three aspects that bring culture and biology together. We need to iron out what is diversity, what is toxicity, and what is optimum.

1. DIVERSITY

Societies do things differently. For example, humans thrive in societies that are monogamous, polygamous, polyandrous and so on. Human societies can be patriarchal or matriarchal. In some societies men take care of babies; in others they don't. Just because we do marriage, it doesn't mean that is the 'ultimate' or the only way to be in a society. There is no one right way when it comes to human beings, unlike the other primates. And I'm sure there is no one right way when it comes to birth. There are lots of different ways in which humans birth their babies.

2. TOXICITY

Cultures can be toxic, and humans can survive them. We are a diverse species, and we are also a resilient species. For example, Chinese foot-binding is a toxic way to treat the mind and body. During the many years that this was in practice, the population survived, with not much consideration for the long-term effects on families. When it comes to babies, we know that colostrum is very healthy for a baby, and that to stop the baby from getting it is risking the welfare of the baby. Yet many cultures have practices which inhibit the chances of the baby getting colostrum, ours included. With birth, women can birth in toxic environments, and still survive. However, the fallout emotionally and physically, for both the woman and the baby, has only provoked research interest in the last few years.

3. OPTIMAL PRACTICES

Despite the fact that there are many different ways to birth, and that societies do things in a toxic way, it is also true that there are optimal environments and basic needs for humans, which, when met, will help us to thrive. For example, people need to interact with each other to be physically and mentally healthy. People need to have loving interactions as babies and children to grow into functional adults. People need a range of vitamins and minerals to stay healthy. The things that we need to thrive are not obvious, and science and psychology work hard to try to isolate the things that help us be optimally healthy. This is very much the case with regard to birth.

The job of psychology is to understand what is toxic to us. We can then begin to understand why we become sick, or why we hurt and kill each other, or why we become depressed and anxious. If we can understand what is toxic about birth, we can understand why trauma following childbirth seems to be on the rise, and what we can do about it. Psychology is also interested in what helps us to thrive. Psychology is interested in why we experience satisfaction, joy, contentment, love, peace and harmony. This applies to birth, as it seems to be the case that some women come away from their births feeling amazing, feeling complete and satisfied, feeling strong, powerful and invincible. A great birth is arguably a great foundation from which to begin the challenging job of transforming into fully fledged parents. Parents need to learn to fall in love with their baby, to enjoy the baby, and to forgive themselves for not being perfect, and so on. It is important to know how we can help parents to thrive through birth, rather than just survive birth. This book may help you understand why birth was an ordeal for you, and help you to come to terms with the disappointment or anger or horror or shame or flashbacks associated with having had a difficult birth.

BIRTH AS NATURE KNOWS IT

Birth is a physiological event that happens to all mammals, not just humans. It is something our bodies are designed to do, in the same way as digesting our food, or going to sleep, or going to the toilet are. It has become a bit of a cliché to say 'your body is designed to birth a baby'; so much so, that I think it isn't really understood what we mean by that. Our modern society certainly hasn't got the message, because it is behaving as if the last thing it ever expects to happen is for a baby to be born spontaneously and naturally. It is something that we seem to have lost sight of. In our modern world, birth has become synonymous with hospitals, procedures, doctors, pain, ordeals, classes, education, expertise and danger.

I was at a birth where, just after the baby was born, the father turned to me astounded, and said 'The baby just came out!' I smiled and congratulated him. He repeated it. 'But the baby just came out!' I said yes, it's lovely isn't it? And he said it again. 'I can't believe the baby just came out!' I then said 'What did you expect to happen?' And he said 'I don't know'. I have even heard birth be compared to having your teeth removed. However, it doesn't take much grey matter to work out that birth is more akin to taking a bowel movement, than it is to having your teeth extracted. This is because your body is programmed to do it, and it will do it even if you don't try, or

mother and a live baby. We are lucky enough in ou
to be able to focus on thriving, not just surviving,
about the things that I see all the time as a bi
The love, ecstasy, joy, empowerment and
comes with a good birth. Yes, you rea
often enjoy birth. I hear them tell
again in a heartbeat because they
feelings of immense love, joy
sorry to labour this point, b
painful to hear if you ha
devastated. This will
sense that your b
dealing with a
Underst
us to un
that

ways in different societies. Some with partners present, some without, some with toddlers around, some without, some in a hospital, some at home, some with drugs, some without, some standing up, some lying down, some in peace and quiet, some in noise and bustle. All well and good. As for point two, we want to understand the circumstances that can make birth toxic. Why do so many women come away from their births feeling emotionally wretched, devastated, humiliated, like a failure, or broken? Is this to be expected? Is it the case that we need to try to survive birth, in the same way that we may survive a car crash, or a driving test? Is it part of the human condition to experience birth as an ordeal? No. I don't think so. The third part is to understand how we can thrive at birth – how, as human beings, we can optimally birth babies. And I don't just mean 'survive'. I'm not just talking about a live

r society
I am talking
th companion.
exhilaration that
d that right. Women
e that they would do it
enjoyed it. Women describe
and ecstasy as they birth. I'm
because I understand that it can be
ve come away from your birth feeling
be especially true if you had an intuitive
rth could have been amazing, and you are
sense of grief around that.

nding good birth, as well as bad birth, can help
derstand *why* you might feel so devastated by the fact
you didn't get a lovely birth. We are only just beginning
understand the physiology of the birthing mother. The
structure of her body, her vagina, her pelvis, her clitoris,
her hormones, and how all those change as she births. The
ignorance on this subject has been, and continues to be,
monumental. In fact, it's not very different to the monumental
ignorance that was endemic 200 years ago around sex and
women in Victorian society. Let me elaborate.

A VICTORIAN VIEW OF WOMEN AND SEX

In order to highlight what I am saying, I want to tell you a story
which illustrates some struggles that women had in Victorian
Britain. It goes like this:

In the Victorian era, a husband's conjugal rights were
a wife's conjugal duty. Sexual intercourse for women was
viewed as at best boring, and at worst unpleasant and painful.
It was regarded as 'undignified' and 'unladylike'. Imagine for
a moment, how a young Victorian woman might have felt on
her wedding night. She knows that something rather odd is
expected of her tonight – but she doesn't really know what it

will be, or what it will be like. Her mother is evidently happy for her, but also rather anxious on her behalf. Her mother has given her some advice, along the lines of 'as long as your husband is gentle, you will be all right'. Goodness – what if he isn't? Mother also says that there may well be blood on the sheets, and it will hurt. That really is rather worrying, but she is reassured that it is always worse the first time, and after that things start to get easier. The best piece of advice that people seem to be able to give is to 'lie back and think of England, and it will be okay'. It would seem that a Victorian lady should endure it, and wait for it to be over.

Now, we know that in Victorian Britain people had not really grasped that ladies have a sexual response cycle, or that they could become aroused, or that they could find sex desirable (of course, some women and some men had grasped this – but on a cultural level, it wasn't understood). The fact that a woman could release hormones associated with arousal and enjoyment of sexual intercourse was not understood. Orgasms were a male domain, and the clitoris was, frankly, viewed as problematic.

So, let us go back to the bride on her wedding night, and the advice of her mother. The young lady would go to her wedding bed feeling anxious, worried, and unsure. You do not need science or psychology to tell you that this will affect her ability to relax and enjoy the occasion. She will lie there, worrying, tensing up, flinching when he touches her, waiting for it to be over, and as a result will not release the right hormones for sexual arousal. Sexual arousal and penetration are inhibited by anxiety and fear. Many marriages of the time were annulled because they were never consummated. And they weren't consummated because the act of sexual intercourse was apparently impossible! The woman's body refused to work, and penetration could not occur.

These physical problems with penetration didn't exist because there was anything wrong with women's bodies, they existed because of the psychology of the woman – the fear surrounding the whole process of sexual intercourse. If women were actually able to 'perform' sexual intercourse, it was often painful or traumatic. Much of what we know about Victorian sexual experiences comes from letters that were written at the time. Emily Austin, for example, described her first sexual experience as 'a nightmare of physical pain'.

Hopefully, you can already see the analogy I'm making between sex in Victorian times and birth in modern times. How often do we hear birth described like this nowadays? I believe that birth is in the same place now that sex for women was back then. When a woman becomes pregnant, she is told that birth is at best bearable and at worst traumatic – but always painful. There is a lot of ignorance about the biology of birthing a baby, and even more ignorance about the psychology of birthing a baby. She might be reassured that birth is in good hands these days, that the hospital saves lives, and that as long as she can have an epidural she will be okay. Due to fear and sterile environments and birth attendants she has never met before, she does not release the cocktail of hormones necessary for birth to unfold as nature intended. On the contrary, tension or anxiety releases hormones that inhibit spontaneous birth and labour, which makes for a longer, more painful, and more dangerous birth, with a much greater chance of intervention. Society's view that birth is painful, scary and not in the least bit pleasant turns out to be true.

But the Victorians were wrong about women and sex. We now know that women can and do enjoy sexual intercourse, and that it can be an amazing experience (and an awful one too). Whether it is amazing or awful depends upon a number of things – but primarily on her willingness, relaxation and trust during the process. Are we making the same mistake with women and birthing that was being made about women and sex so many years ago? Well, yes. It seems that birth, like sex, can be enjoyable or awful, and that which way it goes depends upon the woman's willingness, relaxation and who she is with during the process. If you don't believe this, it is because you have never entertained the idea before. Now that it is occurring to you for the first time, start to take a new look at the evidence around you. There is plenty out there.

Midwives, mothers, fathers, journalists, and film-makers, are all starting to talk about ecstatic births. There are books, films, DVDs, amazing clips on social media, stories from The Farm in Tennessee – all featuring women in modern society birthing quickly and easily. I mention modern society, because we've all heard the stories about African women working in fields stopping to birth their babies upright, and then walking on with their babies. It would seem that in industrialised society women are starting to do the same, but they are talking about not only how easy it can be, but how ecstatic and empowering it can be too. Wow, what a well-kept secret! The difference isn't in our bodies, but in our culture.

HOW WE DO IT IN WESTERN MODERN SOCIETIES

You might like to think that you are your own individual with your own independent thoughts and beliefs. But I'm afraid that is an illusion. You are actually a product of your society. You couldn't have learnt to speak English fluently and seamlessly if you hadn't been in the society of others speaking English. The television is not enough for children to learn to speak – they need interaction. As you learn your language, you also learn your culture's beliefs and they become so ingrained that it is difficult to tell that it is actually happening.

I am spinning at about 1,000 miles per hour, but I feel as though I am still. We become so accustomed to our assumptions and beliefs that we don't realise they are there. This has been equated to a fish swimming in water. It doesn't even realise that it is in water. It's worth having a think about what messages, assumptions and beliefs you became acculturated to during your upbringing. If it was a Western medicalised culture, I can hazard a guess as to what it might have involved:

It all began when you were old enough to listen to stories, or watch films. So, from as young as about two years old, you were soaking up the narrative of your society. You learned early on in life, through sitcoms, or listening to your mum chat over coffee, or through images of newborn babies in operating theatres, that birth can be an ordeal. You soaked up the messages that birth needs to be in a hospital, where things are done 'to' the mother, and doctors are involved, and there is risk. You learned early in life that birth is potentially dangerous, and needs a doctor to keep both mum and baby alive.

It then carries on. In case you haven't got the message yet that birth is extremely painful, you get shown a film of a woman birthing her baby in a sex education lesson at school. There are bright lights, there are beds, there are doctors, the woman is screaming, and there is blood.

When you are actually pregnant, you get told to go see a midwife, who logs you on as a 'patient' very quickly. You will be told to attend 'appointments', the medical profession will 'monitor' you, 'check' the baby, take bloods, do scans, measure you, tell you what you can and can't do and so you learn to entrust your body to an 'expert' even though you aren't even ill. Meanwhile, you are 'invited' for blood tests, you and your baby are screened for a long list of potential dangers: are you and your baby the right weight, correct bump size, are your blood measurements normal, are your blood sugars normal, should you be this fat or round at this point, and so on and so on. Numbers and figures are applied to you throughout the pregnancy. You are even given a 'due date' as if such a thing actually exists. It does not, by the way. Babies aren't like cakes in an oven. You don't wait 22 minutes for a 'ping' and then remove the cake. Babies are like apples on a tree. They are ripe around September. Some are ripe quicker than others. You can't predict which one will be ripe first. You can't force it to be ripe any quicker.

When you aren't at your patient appointments, you hear other people's warnings and horror stories of their births. They are frightening. You attend 'classes' to learn how to have a baby. You learn that movement in labour is good. You learn that breathing can 'help'. You are warned that you might end up in theatre with 10 people in the room if there's an emergency. You learn what forceps look like. You learn that you will probably need pain relief. You don't feel all that much better.

When you finally do go into labour, the hospital tells you to stay at home as long as possible, and that they don't actually want to see you or help you anyway. This is confusing. If you insist on coming in, they do a 'check' (put their fingers into your vagina and have a good feel) and tell you that you are wrong, you aren't in labour yet. You go home. A little despondent. A little distressed. You come back in, they do another 'check' and then they 'allow' you into a brightly lit room with instruments and machines dotted about, and you are left there. Or, they ask you to lie on the bed (hang on, didn't all those antenatal classes talk about the benefits of movement and being upright????), wire you up to a machine that makes you paranoid about your baby's heartbeat, and then leave the room again. You begin to settle in. A few hours later, your nice midwife tells you her shift is over. You are introduced to another midwife. I could go on, and I could really have some fun with the pushing stage, but I think you've read enough!

Everything about the above scenario reinforces the idea that birth is a painful ordeal that you must try to survive at best, and endure at worst. It has the effect of frightening us, which has the effect of making pregnancy and birth more dangerous. Physiologically, it's not all that different to other natural bodily functions, such as falling asleep, or going to the toilet, or having an orgasm. We do need the right environment to do it in. Here are my top five modern faux pas that your body was not evolved for, and which make birthing a baby more difficult.

FAUX PAS 1: YOUR BODY HAS NOT EVOLVED TO BIRTH WELL WHEN IT DOESN'T FEEL SAFE

A woman is particularly vulnerable during and just after the birth of her baby (just try to imagine running away with a newborn baby attached to your insides via an umbilical cord!). For that reason, nature designed us to not birth when we don't feel safe. It's similar to sleeping. We are vulnerable when we sleep too, and it is much harder to get to sleep when we don't feel safe, or we feel anxious. Both birthing and sleeping involve release of the sleep hormone, melatonin. If you are nervous or frightened it won't flow so well.

FAUX PAS 2: YOUR BODY HAS NOT EVOLVED TO BIRTH WELL IN A BRIGHTLY LIT ROOM

There are a few environmental factors which make it more difficult for any mammal to birth a baby without medical intervention, and one of those factors is light. Most labours begin at night, for humans and for diurnal mammals alike. As mentioned above, melatonin is released when we sleep. Daylight and artificial light reduce melatonin production. We labour and birth better in the dark. Unfortunately, this biological fact has not been taken into account in most hospital environments. Arguably, it is regarded as more important that the environment is suitable for the doctor, than it is for the labouring mother.

FAUX PAS 3: YOUR BODY HAS NOT EVOLVED TO BIRTH WELL WITH SOMEONE WHO ISN'T NURTURING YOU

When a woman is in the process of birth, she is vulnerable simply because she cannot run or fight back. She needs people around her who will do the fighting and protecting on her behalf. She needs someone who has her back, who likes and respects her. In our maternity system, the midwife supporting her at her most vulnerable time is usually a stranger. We are not evolved to relax deeply and fully when faced with a stranger – even if the stranger is a qualified midwife and is very nice indeed.

FAUX PAS 4: YOUR BODY HAS NOT EVOLVED TO BIRTH WELL WHEN IN AN UNFAMILIAR PLACE

If you think that an unfamiliar place has no effect on you, think again. When I run my two-day workshops, I can't tell you where people will sit on the first day, other than to say they will sit with someone that they already know. But I can tell you where everyone will sit on the second day. This is because they will almost always sit in the same place! We like familiarity, it helps us feel secure. If I shake things up by moving the chairs, there's always quite a bit of consternation and unease.

FAUX PAS 5: BIRTH IS NOT A SPORTING EVENT: YOU CAN'T DO IT BETTER BY TRYING HARDER

Birth is not like running a marathon. It is not like taking an exam. It is not about your stamina, or your planning, or your resilience, or your assertiveness, or your motherliness, or any of that. Birth is more like drifting off to sleep, or digesting your food or recovering from a cold. You can't 'try harder' to drift off to sleep; it won't work. You just give your body the right environment and it'll do it. Sleep needs quiet and warmth, digestion needs rest and good food, recovery from a cold needs the same. If a medical issue develops, such as insomnia, or Crohn's disease or pneumonia, then you get help from a doctor. But you don't blame yourself for not trying harder. It's the same for birth.

Research is quite clear that there is one really important point about normal physiological processes, and that is that we do need the right environment. Our society is failing to realise this, which is leading to a lot of difficult births and a lot of women blaming their own bodies when it goes wrong. But in fact, all that their bodies did was to respond to an environment which was not ideal for birth. One which was not conducive to feeling safe, secure, familiar, unhurried, dark and peaceful.

BIRTH PHILOSOPHIES: BIRTH TRAUMA AND THE MEDICAL MODEL OF BIRTH

Are you aware of the difference between a midwife and an obstetrician? They can be very similar, in that they are both trained in pregnancy and birth, and they are both a professional presence, assisting in the birth of babies. They both have the mother and the baby's lives in their hands. However, that is where the similarities end. They can be seen to be worlds apart in terms of their philosophy and practice when it comes to assisting births. As Sheila Stubbs put it:

'The midwife considers the miracle of childbirth as normal, and leaves it alone unless there's trouble. The obstetrician normally sees childbirth as trouble; if he leaves it alone, it's a miracle.'

Historically, there has always been a power struggle between doctors and midwives, ever since doctors began to be involved in the birthing room in the second half of the last millennium. Before then, attending births was the job of women only, and midwives in particular. They used folklore, experience, passed-down wisdom, and herbs to do their job. (These herbs included ergot, which was used by midwives throughout the Middle Ages to assist labour. Its modern derivative is the drug ergometrine, used widely in modern maternity services.)

Male doctors began to become interested in birthing, and with their endowed status, formal education, and tools such as forceps, they began to take over the birthing room a few hundred years ago. One of the ways that this happened was that attendance at a birth by unqualified midwives was banned, and women were banned from becoming qualified. Forceps were introduced, epitomising to some extent the power struggle that was born in the birthing room. On the one hand, forceps were praised as a blessing that saved lives, as illustrated by this Wikipedia statement:

'The introduction of the obstetrical forceps provided huge advances in the medicalisation of childbirth.'

Others believe that the use of forceps represents an inhumane and violent obstetric practice, and there have been calls to ban them. As one obstetrician put it:

'Forceps are a great instrument to use for the obstetrician but it's very much at the cost of the woman.'

I am talking about birthing philosophies and culture here, not about people as individuals. At a risk of stereotyping and caricaturing a complex subject, I am interested in two main models of childbirth which are relevant to the current state of birth in our society. A patriarchal, medical model on the one hand, and a feminine, midwifery model on the other. The medical model tends to assume that birth is precarious, it needs medical equipment and qualified staff and drugs and hospitals, and it needs to be timed and monitored and measured. The birthing woman comes in and has stuff done to her by professionals in order to facilitate the birth of the baby. It's not much different from a patient coming in for a medical procedure or an operation – the doctor is the one who knows what he or she is doing. The baby would not be born without the doctor there. This is the model that is most prevalent in our social media.

In contrast, a midwifery model tends to assume that birth works well in its natural form, that the mother knows intuitively how to birth her baby, that birth should be respected and left well alone, that it shouldn't be rushed or timed, that medical procedures can inhibit or endanger the birthing process, and that the baby can be trusted to be born without interference. The role of the birth professional is akin to that of a lifeguard – a lifeguard does not wade in and hold the swimmer up in the water, moving their arms and legs for them. The lifeguard watches carefully from the sidelines, and only wades in when there are sure signs of trouble. They then call a doctor if they need to do more than on-site first aid.

The midwifery model is one which, I believe, a lot of women align themselves to intuitively. I hear a lot of women come to me saying 'I don't want medical intervention, I want to be left alone in labour, I feel that if I was at home, undisturbed, I would have an amazing birth, I am scared of them doing stuff to me that I don't want' and so on.

This was certainly the case for me. As soon as I knew I was pregnant, I knew I wanted a natural birth. I genuinely do not know where this came from. It seemed to come from somewhere intuitive. I wanted a home birth. I did not know anyone who had had a home birth, I had never been interested in how women birth, or the culture of birth. My mother had her babies in hospital – there was no reason that I know of why it was so important to me to have a home birth. But it was.

I went on to have two babies at home and one in hospital. After the hospital birth, my husband summed up our experience like this: 'When you birth at home, the midwives are invited attendants at your birth. When you birth in a hospital, you are their patient'.

In my work as a birth doula, I see this again and again. Women at home, birthing with midwives in attendance, are much more likely to be honoured, empowered and respected.

Women birthing in hospital under the care of doctors are much more likely to be belittled, not listened to, bullied into 'consenting', and threatened. It is no wonder that women are wary of the medical model, and caught between the belief that they need a hospital to stay safe, and being scared of having their dignity and power taken from them in the process.

The difference between a midwifery model of birth and a medicalised model of birth can also be seen in the use of language. Language is important, because it is necessarily emotive: it evokes emotion. For example, the words 'slim' and 'skinny' mean the same, but don't feel the same. Words are powerful, in that they guide a person's experience and formation of assumptions and beliefs. Words which I hear commonly in terms of birth include the use of the phrase 'emergency caesarean section', to mean an unscheduled caesarean section. Most unscheduled caesarean sections are less of an emergency, and more of a change of plan. For example, sometimes, it is the case that during labour, a woman 'fails to progress' (note the language there) and labour is going slowly, and the medics think that it would be safer to go to surgery to avoid mum getting exhausted and bleeding, or baby getting compromised, so the decision is often made to go to theatre instead of carry on with the original plan of a vaginal delivery. This is not really an 'emergency'. It's a change of plan. I know that emergency sections do happen, though quite rarely. They are known as 'crash c-sections' which is also rather emotive! I really don't want one of those, thank you very much!

Medical language around childbirth reflects the narrative of medicalised birth – that birth is precarious, that a woman needs help and intervention, that things are done to her and so on. Think about the following words: 'failure to progress', 'the midwife delivered the baby', 'you're not allowed', 'how often are the pains', 'you are low risk'.

I'd like to make a quick aside, which I always feel that I

have to include, in case I upset the sensitivities of the current patriarchy too much. There are plenty of men, and male and female doctors who subscribe to the midwifery model, and there are plenty of women and men, and male midwives who subscribe to the medical model. This is not about individuals; it is about culture, attitudes, beliefs and practices. Likewise, there are home births under midwife care that are disrespectful and coercive, and there are hospital births that are peaceful and honoured and wonderful.

Furthermore, I am not against doctors and the medical system being involved in birth. Doctors save lives. Medicine saves lives. My point is simply that we don't need a lifeguard in order to stay alive in the water, we don't need an ambulance in order to drive a car, and we don't need a doctor to birth a baby. Lifeguards, ambulances and doctors should be on standby, to be called in if, and only if, things go wrong. The World Health Organization is quite clear that medical over-involvement in birth may compromise the health of mother and baby.

Some women choose a medicalised birth, while some want a natural birth. The research is clear that in order to reduce distress after birth, all women, no matter what type of birth they choose, need to be listened to and respected. In our medicalised system, power and control in the birthing room matters in terms of reducing birth trauma. Many of the women I've worked with feel traumatised by issues around power in the birthing room. They describe feeling as though they were not listened to, or that they were belittled, or that things were done to them without their consent, or that they were coerced or rushed, or bullied.

Research suggests that reducing unnecessary obstetric intervention can prevent trauma, not only for mothers, but also for midwives (Creedy & Gamble). It matters that we allow women to birth with dignity, power and honour, throughout the process of birth, regardless of what they wished for, or what turn their birthing took.

THE DARK SIDE OF BIRTH:
OBSTETRIC VIOLENCE AND BIRTH RAPE

❗ *Trigger warning: reference to sexual violence, traumatic*
● *births and obstetric violence throughout remaining chapter.*

I'm going back to sex as an analogy for birth. Earlier, I made a comparison between Victorian views of sex and modern views of childbirth. I am now going to make a comparison between attitudes associated with what has been termed 'rape culture' and current attitudes towards obstetric practices.

Rape culture is a sociological term, which describes the idea that societal attitudes and beliefs in our society about rape contribute to the normalising of sexual violence, and the way that we do or don't address the problem of rape. Our society's attitudes are changing, thank goodness. For example, not so long ago, it was mainstream belief that women couldn't be raped by their husbands, and this was enshrined in law. It is becoming better understood that there are pervasive problems for women in finding justice. Often, victims are not believed. There is even a term for it, which makes me wince: 'cry rape'.

The list of problems for women in being properly respected and heard when they report sexual assault goes on and on. They are told they made it up, imagined it, brought it upon themselves, shouldn't have worn those clothes, shouldn't have got drunk, shouldn't have flirted, that they deserved it, that he was enticed, that he couldn't help himself, that he got mixed messages, that she needs punishing, that she enjoyed it, that she's over-reacting, that it was no big deal, that it was unimportant, that she should have fought back. Thankfully, society's attitudes are changing for the better. You only need to spend a little time watching television from a few decades ago to see the differences. The impact of society's attitudes towards rape is such that the 'alleged' victims often carry the burden of shame, guilt, anxiety and confusion.

In my clinic, what I see when I work with women who have

been traumatised at their birth, is that they also feel shame, guilt, anxiety and confusion. They feel they should have said something, been more assertive, got angry, not made a fuss, not got upset and so on. Why is this? Is it similar?

You may or may not have come across the terms 'birth rape' or 'obstetric rape' or 'obstetric violence'. It is a contentious phrase, and while you may or may not agree with the terminology, the fact remains that many women come away from their births feeling as though they have been raped. In this excerpt, Shea Richland helps us see why many women want the term birth rape to be recognised:

> 'My daughter's birth contained all the elements of a rape. I was taken to a strange place and told what to do. My clothes and personal possessions were taken from me. I was forced into an uncomfortable position and bound. I was threatened (it's hospital policy, don't make trouble). I was drugged and knocked unconscious... My vagina was cut and a man's tool (forceps) was inserted into my body. I was robbed. That which was most precious to me, my baby, was taken from me. All this was done against my will.' (Shea Richland, retired midwife and childbirth educator, *Midwifery Today*, 'Birth rape, another midwife's story')

There is a growing recognition and awareness that some of the beliefs and assumptions around medical practices in the labour ward are not dissimilar to those outdated 'rape culture' beliefs about sexual practices in bedrooms/at parties that we strive so hard to eliminate. For example, it is currently mainstream belief that women can't be assaulted by their obstetricians, and that they should allow him or her to do what they need to do. It is okay to regularly have fingers and instruments put into your vagina, it is okay to be told to lie on your back and have your legs strapped into stirrups, it is okay to be told to be quiet and let the doctor do what they need to do, it is okay to be intimately poked and prodded by a person whose name you don't even know, and who doesn't know yours, and to be told to 'leave your dignity at the door' and so on. These aspects of obstetric 'care' are normalised.

If you do an internet search for birth and take a look at the images, you will see what I mean. A woman in stirrups in a hospital gown will be there. Being put on your back with your legs akimbo is normalised. And yet no woman that I have ever met has said 'Oh yes, I liked the stirrups, I felt safe with them, I felt like I could push more easily, I felt protected and less vulnerable'.

On the contrary, I have heard many women say that being made to lie on their back during labour was awful, and that they protested, but they were told it was necessary. I have heard countless stories of women telling me that they said 'no' but that the staff persisted anyway. I have heard stories of women saying that they felt verbally threatened when they didn't consent. I have heard women tell me that it is 'odd' because they almost feel as though they have been sexually assaulted – even though they haven't. I have heard women tell me that they felt as though the doctors treated them 'like a carrier bag. They got the goods out, and then left me'.

I am not alone in hearing these stories. As a birth doula myself, I am part of the birth doula community. Doulas are people who are an emotional support for women in labour. The things we witness in the birthing room leave us with our own little scars too. Midwives and doctors also watch obstetric brutality. In one study, the distress of watching women be dehumanised and have their choices taken from them was one of the main factors contributing to midwife burnout (Patterson). Just one small sentence, which birth professionals hear regularly, can have a devastating impact on the mother. I call it 'playing the dead baby card'. It is a form of coercion and control, which Paula's story illustrates.

PAULA'S STORY

Paula came to me for help for birth trauma when her baby was 8 months old. She had tried to get help but was still struggling. She told me that she had been 'mistreated by one obstetrician', and was having nightmares two to three times a week. She told me that on her darkest days, she had planned her own suicide, because she simply didn't want to be here anymore. This is despite the fact that she loved her baby very deeply. She told me that every time she has to go back to the hospital for health checks, she gets panic attacks. She told me that she had been told she was depressed. But she did not think she was depressed. She thought she had been traumatised.

She told me her birth story. There was so much more to her story than the verbal assault by the obstetrician, as is often the case. She had simply not been listened to properly by midwives, doctors, therapists and obstetricians throughout her pregnancy and labour. She is a highly educated scientific researcher. She is very gentle and soft-spoken and rather lovely. I've often wondered if youth and/or femininity increase your chances of being mistreated during labour. Who knows?

Paula had had a beautiful start to her labour. She had laboured at home, with her husband, dancing through the contractions to music that they both loved, her hormones steadily climbing, with her feeling more empowered and awash with the love hormones associated with labour. Unfortunately, after she went into hospital, her beautiful labour was brought to a halt. In fact, the way that she was treated in hospital caused her to develop PTSD.

Upon admission to the hospital, Paula was categorised as high risk because she was labouring just before the 37-week window of 'full term'. She tried to explain that her due dates had never been right, and this had been in her notes all along, because she had raised the issue numerous times. It was written that she 'claims' her due dates are wrong, but then this 'claim' was ignored. She was still taken to the doctor-led unit rather than midwife-led. Fast forward now to the moment when the obstetrician came in. Paula knew she was close to delivering her baby. She knew she wanted to focus on the birth, take her energy inwards, and birth her baby in a calm way to reduce the chances of tearing, and also to fully savour this special moment in her life. The obstetrician told her the baby needed to be monitored with an electronic foetal monitor (EFM). Paula declined, saying 'I don't need it, my baby is not at risk'. She could already feel the baby's head between her legs.

Now, it is an offence to touch a woman in labour without her consent. So how did they get consent? The obstetrician said to her 'If you don't have it (EFM), your baby may die'. Those words, words which are spoken so often that doctors don't really think about it, and doulas like me call it 'playing the dead baby card', had a dramatic effect on Paula. She sobbed to me 'Those words really *hurt me. I would never do* anything *that would kill my baby. After what he said, I would have agreed to* anything'.

As a result, Paula was in a panic, scared, confused, and she pushed so hard that her baby came out far too quickly, causing a great deal of perineal damage and dangerous blood loss for Paula. Paula described this obstetrician as having attacked her, as having violated her human rights. Not only had she been violated, but she had had 'something beautiful taken from me' – the opportunity to welcome her baby in a gentle and loving way.

And I agree. But I'm not sure many others would, because the narrative in our system does not allow it. This was evidenced in the therapy she had been offered on the NHS before coming to me for help. While trying to explain to her therapist what had happened and why she had been traumatised, her therapist remarked 'Would you rather have a consultant that treats you well, or one that does his job?'

Paula has since looked into the option of suing the doctor, but she has been told by lawyers that it would be her word against his, and because her baby isn't dead or injured, it would be almost impossible to win. This is all part of a system that doesn't understand the damage it is doing to women, that doesn't listen to women, that is robbing women of their birth rights. I'm glad to say that Paula and her baby are doing just fine now. No more nightmares. She can tell her story without crying. Her husband says she's happy again. She told me it was life-changing – just 'wow'. She only needed three sessions of trauma treatment, because there was nothing wrong with her. She was just reacting normally to having been treated appallingly.

If we fail to acknowledge that obstetric violence is real, we silence women. Language is implicitly bound up in attitudes, assumptions, thinking and culture. If people come away from birth feeling as if they have been a victim of obstetric rape, and there is not common language to frame what happened, where do they go with that narrative? Women come away confused about their feelings, unable to tell their story, and blaming themselves. They feel that they should be grateful because their baby is alive. That the way they were treated shouldn't matter. That doctors are powerful because they are trained and knowledgeable and shouldn't be questioned.

I am a therapist who specialises in birth trauma, and I can't name one person who did not feel guilty about the fact that their birth was awful. Women blame themselves. 'I should have said no, I should have been more assertive, I should have written a birth plan, I should never have written a birth plan, I should have had a home birth, I should have planned a c-section, I should have got angry, I should have researched more beforehand, I shouldn't have been so trusting'… and so on. None of this was their fault. These women were treated badly by a system that took control, took the power, belittled and put them down, interfered physically, sexually and brutally, and yet they are left feeling to blame.

When they complain, they are told 'the doctor saved your life, all birth is brutal, what did you expect, be grateful that you have a healthy baby' and so on.

I am so sorry if you are one of the women who have experienced this first hand. You are not alone. You are not the only one who struggles to understand why you feel like you do, who struggles to be heard, or to be believed, or to be understood. Society would have you believe that because you have a healthy baby, you should be grateful, and you should stop moaning. The effect of this is that you don't tell people, and you end up being the one who carries the burden of the confusion, the shame, the guilt, the anxiety, and the trauma.

I said it at the beginning of the book, and I'll say it again. If you were treated unkindly or brutally, this is not your fault. It's not your shame or blame to bear. You have the compassion and understanding of many doulas, many midwives, many obstetricians. Many people who know the system, know that it needs to change. And one of those changes is to acknowledge that obstetric violence and birth rape is real, and it might have happened to you.

BIRTH AND STRUCTURAL RACISM

While I don't want to add to the hysteria around birth being dangerous, I do want to share one statistic which is alarming. Even though perinatal maternal mortality is very low indeed in the West, it is still the case that a woman of colour is five times more likely to die as a result of having a baby in Britain, and three to four times more likely to die perinatally in the USA than a white woman.

Jennie Joseph, an expert in this area, is clear that the reasons are to do with structural racism, rather than anything physiologically different about black women's bodies. She has highlighted one major way in which women of colour are treated differently in the perinatal period, and how this affects outcomes. And it is to do with not being listened to.

The well-documented case of Serena Williams illustrates the point very well. Soon after the birth of her baby daughter, this famous, wealthy, admired, powerful tennis player fell prey to being disregarded and not listened to. In this case, it could have cost her life, and it did lead to days and days of extensive medical care. According to an interview she gave with *Vogue* magazine, her story goes like this:

SERENA WILLIAMS WASN'T LISTENED TO

Ms Williams was in her postnatal room with her own mother, one day after the birth of her baby. Ms Williams began to have sensations of breathlessness. Her instinct told her that this was a sign of a pulmonary embolism, and that she needed an IV with heparin, which is a blood thinner. Ms Williams had a history of blood clots, so she knew the signs and the treatment necessary. She stepped outside of her room and calmly told a nurse of her symptoms, adding that she needed an IV with a blood thinner, and a CT scan to check for clots. According to *Vogue* magazine, the nurse disregarded her, thinking she was confused. (Yep, you read that right. *Confused*. I was shocked when I read this.) So Ms Williams 'insisted', as you would if you were scared that your life was at risk. At her insistence, the doctor was called. I do wonder what might have happened if a very young, non-famous African-American woman who lives in relative poverty had 'insisted'. Anyhow, the doctor who was called *also* disregarded what she was saying, by scanning her legs with a doppler instead of ordering a CT scan on her lungs. This is odd, given that her symptoms were breathing difficulties, and I don't know of anyone who has breathing difficulties in their legs. Ms Williams repeated that she needed a CT scan and heparin. The ultrasound revealed nothing, and she finally underwent a CT scan, which showed several small blood clots in her lungs. She was immediately put on the heparin drip. As I say, this led to a host of ensuing medical emergencies and complications.

As far as I know, the staff concerned were not reprimanded. In a structurally racist system, the racism would not even have been recognised, never mind acted upon. And reading this, you might even be thinking 'No, I can't believe that happened just because she was a black woman'. In Jennie Joseph's words, 'Serena Williams, [in spite of her] wealth, celebrity, power, agency, she was still in dire straits because she as a black woman… was ignored. This really confirms for us that it is about racism, it's about classism and it's definitely about sexism'. (*Woman's Hour*, Radio 4, 2019)

We don't know how this affected Serena Williams emotionally. She seems to be doing fine now, which makes me happy. If being black makes you more likely to die when you have a baby, and makes you more likely to have a baby prematurely, does it also make you more likely to develop birth trauma? Here's the thing. We have no idea. As far as I know no one has researched it yet. Surprised? Don't be. It's just another example of how being a woman of colour disadvantages you in a system which inherently ignores you at best, and makes dangerous presumptions at worst.

BIRTH AND NOT BEING LISTENED TO

Serena Williams was not listened to after her birth. I hear the same thing all the time from the traumatised women that I work with. As a birth doula, I see it happening a lot too. For example, I remember one birth where the new mother was having stitches after she had birthed. She called out that she wasn't ready because she could feel pain. The doctor ignored her. I had to say 'Stop', get eye contact from the doctor, and to say to her that '[the mother] has asked you to pause because it's hurting her. Did you hear her?' Doing the work that I do, I know anecdotally that not feeling listened to is a contributory factor in the development of birth trauma. This is backed by research looking at the nature of the relationship between mothers and their caregivers. Feeling unsupported is correlated with birth trauma (Ayers). Many of the real-life testimonials that you see in this book involve a sense of not being listened to at some point during the birth. Ruth's traumatic birth was also exacerbated, and might even have been wholly caused, by the experience of not being listened to:

RUTH'S STORY

Ruth came to me for help with birth trauma. You will hear from her again in Chapter 8, and her husband, Mike, shares his story in Chapter 5, on how relatives can help.

The birth had left her with feelings that many mothers will be familiar with after a difficult and medicalised birth. She felt that she had been not listened to, she had lost control, it was partly her fault, and she felt as if she had been assaulted by the staff. The anger and the horror that she felt was directed at herself to some extent, and at the staff to a larger extent. Her traumatic memory involved her feeling that the staff were not listening to her – they were acting without explanation and without her consent.

During therapy, she told me 'my clothes were removed, a hand was put up my vagina, I gave no consent for any of this. I was whisked down a corridor, I needed control at that point, I was yelling 'stop'. People weren't listening. I'm a teacher. When I say stop, children stop!'

The most important thing to her, for personal and spiritual reasons, was for the umbilical cord to remain intact. They cut it immediately and disposed of it, with no regard for Ruth's preferences. She was still unconscious. Later in therapy, when Ruth began to feel much better, and back in control, she would still say, often, 'if only they had TOLD me'. All she needed was for them to explain what was happening while it was happening. An explanation that they needed to remove her clothing because this was now an emergency, an explanation that they needed to put a hand into her vagina to remove the induction pessary, an explanation that a porter was going to whisk her down the corridor as fast as he could because speed mattered at this point, with an explanation that he did not have the jurisdiction to stop the trolley even though she was begging him to. That would have made so much difference to her.

And I know it to be true. Because that traumatic memory had a devastating impact on her psychology. She developed a crippling need to be in control of her life and the people in it. She would get uncontrollable, overwhelming emotion if she felt her husband hadn't listened to her, or people hadn't done what she had told them to do, or done it when she told them to do it. It turns out these overwhelming 'moments' were a form of emotional, or somatic (felt in the body), flashback. I'm pleased to say that she is now recovered following therapy for the trauma.

The impact that 'not being listened to' can have on a woman's feelings after the birth is something that I am very familiar with. What I hear less commonly, is what happened to Ruth when she sought help. Ruth was not listened to by mental health professionals either.

She first got in contact with me four years after the traumatic birth. The first time I spoke to her, she told me she was under the care of a psychiatrist and receiving regular psychotherapy with another therapist. I asked her why she wanted to see me. She said she wanted someone who would treat her birth trauma. I asked her why they couldn't do that. She told me that they wouldn't acknowledge any birth trauma. She told me that although she kept telling them that the problem went back to the birth, they were telling her that the problem lay in her need to be in control (as I outlined above, she was having somatic flashbacks of the birth which were playing out as a horror of not being in control).

She told me 'I know why I'm the way I am. [During the birth] I was saying 'no' to a caesarean section, I lost control, I'm now a control freak. Talking is not treating it. I'm getting *worse'. She had told her psychiatrist this. She had told her psychotherapist this. They didn't listen. Even though her distress was palpable.*

For example, whenever she talked about the devastation of the cord having been cut against her wishes, she became, in her words, 'hysterical'. Despite medication and months of therapy, she was getting worse. In fact, the therapy was actually making it worse, because each time she talked about the birth, she became retraumatised. This is a hazard of counselling or debriefing after a trauma. It can make things worse.

So Ruth came to me for therapy – having looked for a trauma specialist online. It had to be Skype sessions because we were in different countries. After a few sessions focusing on her birth trauma, she started to recover. The recovery was quite dramatic. Towards the end of therapy, Ruth made me laugh when she told me that she wanted this book to be printed in hardback. I asked why. She said 'Because when I get a copy, I'm going to go into the clinic and I'm going to hit them [her previous psychiatrist and therapist] over the head with it. That should help them to get the message that birth trauma is a thing'.

Of course she was right: unless a woman is actively psychotic, it seems to me that she is almost always right about her own needs and emotional state. And even if she is actively psychotic, she still needs to be listened to.

SOCIETIES THAT BREAK WOMEN: FGM, FOOT-BINDING AND INSTITUTIONALISED BIRTH ABUSE

I've watched *Horrible Histories* with my sons for years. I love that programme. It is very funny. It highlights to us the craziness of the things we used to believe, especially with regard to medicine. It is as though that no longer happens.

As though we never do crazy things in this society any more. Crazy things that societies do often involve debilitating treatment of girls and women.

I've often wondered about societies which normalise abuse of female bodies, such as the culturalised practice of female genital mutilation (FGM), which impacts girls' ability to develop sexually. Or the practice of Chinese foot-binding, which affects girls' ability to walk and run properly. I often wonder what the effect is psychologically. Of course, there is an element of physical control involved (control of sexuality and freedom of movement), but there is also an element of damaging the psyche, the spirit, so that a patriarchal society can avoid the threat of feminine power. And I feel that the way we birth in our society is not very different.

We tell girls to fear it from an early age, we tell them they can't do it, it's torturous, they'll need doctors and hospitals, they're wrong if they want a c-section and they're ridiculous if they plan for a natural birth, and then we strap them on their backs under strip lighting with a stranger or two, and pull out their baby with instruments or wheel them to theatre to 'save' them when they 'couldn't' do it naturally.

When they come out of it broken, we tell them that at least they have a healthy baby and the doctor saved them. What impact does this have on the female psyche? How different is our society to the ones that believe in FGM and foot-binding?

There is a whole other conversation to be had about the damage done to babies too – taking their colostrum, taking them from their mothers by ritualising the cutting of the cord, then separating them in ritualised beliefs that babies should sleep alone, making breastfeeding so difficult in our society, telling mothers to let them 'cry it out' when they are communicating their distress at being left alone... and so on. The opportunity to feel empowered and powerful and untouchable and forceful and proud and deeply strong and in love with their baby is taken from mothers. This is all regarded as normal and sane in our society. I regard it as insane and damaging to the female psyche in much the same way as FGM and Chinese foot-binding have been. There. I said it.

LISTEN WITH MOTHER: BIRTH AS IT SHOULD BE

'Ask the woman, she will tell you everything you need to know'
Ina May Gaskin

I would like peace on earth and the eradication of poverty. I've been told many times that that is a pipe dream, and it goes against human nature. Well so does flying, and we've achieved that with science. I believe that *if* we can ever achieve peace on earth, it is *only* through psychology. Psychology (and sociology) helps us understand greed, violence, aggression, and why we kill each other. It also helps us understand compassion, care-giving, empathy, kindness, sharing and altruism. All these are human nature, and the job of psychology is to understand them better so that we can get closer to knowing what circumstances facilitate those we want to encourage, and what circumstances will minimise those we want to eradicate.

Discoveries and information are coming through so quickly at the moment that I can't keep up with it. These are exciting times, and I firmly believe that the next fifty years or so will see dramatic changes in our understanding and our practice. There are two important areas in terms of making maternity care safer for our psyches. The first concerns the nature of compassion and its relation to health. The second concerns the mind-body connection and the placebo effect. But first, a little about your body's natural birth potential.

BIRTH CAN BE ENJOYABLE: HOW CAN THAT BE?

People don't believe that labour and birth can feel good. They don't know that it has been described by many women as ecstatic, powerful, amazing, addictive. I was a hypnobirthing practitioner and a birth doula for many years, and I heard this a lot from what I read and videos I watched of ecstatic and orgasmic births. But I also heard it from the women that I worked with. Women in towns, villages and cities local to me. Normal, everyday women.

Many times, I was told 'I actually enjoyed it' and 'I would do it again in a heartbeat' and 'if only I could birth again, without having to have another child'. And they didn't just mean the joy of having their baby put in their arms. They meant the whole process: the contractions, the rhythmic flow, the building up, the zoning out, the intensity, the pulsating movements of the baby coming down, the last big stretch and pause before the baby slides out in a rush of adrenaline and joy. With my tongue firmly in my cheek, I would like to ask: how can it be that something, during which the hormones of love, calm and connection (oxytocin and endorphins and melatonin) are abundant, can this feel good? How can it be that something which creates movement and stimulation and pressure on parts of the clitoris which have never been reached before (and parts which have) can feel good? And how is it that after a good deal of striving and effort and physical exertion, we can feel elation like never before, as our goal is reached? What I would really like the answer to, is how our society got to a point where it fails to see that *of course* birth can feel great. How can our society be so incredibly ignorant of female anatomy, that it doesn't even know where the clitoris reaches to, and what happens during birth? How can it be that so many women have been robbed of this experience because society thought that birth was a torturous medical event, not a physiological one?

When you look at the hormones and the physiology involved in birth, it seems obvious that birth can be enjoyable. And if we listen to women who say they enjoyed it, rather than disregard them, disbelieve them or discount them, then we will hear many more women stand up and tell us. At the moment, women keep their stories to themselves, or they are very selective about who they tell and what they share, for fear of being seen to be bragging, or for fear of being disbelieved, or simply thought weird. Let's start listening to women. Surely, understanding what makes for a good birth will inform us when trying to research and understand what makes for a bad or traumatic birth.

THE SOOTHING/COMPASSION SYSTEM: THE KEY TO GOOD HEALTH?

Throughout this book, I refer to the three *systems* of human emotion regulation, which have been developed by Professor Paul Gilbert (see diagram).

From Gilbert, *The Compassionate Mind* (2009).
Reprinted with permission from Little, Brown Book Group.

The fight, flight or freeze system is one of these three systems (termed the 'threat-focused' system by Gilbert), because it has evolved to help us manage emotions and behaviours associated with staying safe and keeping us protected. The systems each incorporate many aspects of our being, such as our physiology, biology, neurology, endocrine system (our hormones), our nervous system, psychology, our emotions, drives, behaviours, thoughts, immune system functioning and more. They are all interlinked, and when our threat-focused system is activated, they all play out together, intertwined, in a connection of worrying thoughts, evasive actions, anxious feelings, release of specific hormones and the powering up of specific brain regions. When we feel scared or anxious during birth, this system fires up as an evolved mechanism for self-protection. We get scared. Or angry. Or both. After the birth, when it is all over, the brain sometimes carries on activating the threat system, leaving us feeling scared and angry even though we no longer need to protect ourselves. This happens when we have been traumatised.

The second system outlined by Gilbert is the drive system or the incentive/resource-focused system. This is associated with getting things done and being motivated and excited by life, and it has evolved to make sure we eat, mate, and succeed in life in general. When this system is activated, specific regions of the brain fire up, specific hormones are released, the body is energised, and our thoughts and emotions are all in sync with the goal of getting something done or achieving something. It's quite a nice feeling (unlike the threat-focused system which generally feels awful).

The third system is the one that is relevant to this chapter. It is key to reducing birth trauma, and to making birth a better experience for health professionals, for mothers, for families and for babies. This is the soothing/affiliative/connected focused system, which has evolved to facilitate the care-taking that is so inherent in humanity. Babies, children and adults need each other to survive and to thrive. We depend upon the mammalian care-taking system that involves nurturing, protecting, feeding, sheltering, reassuring, co-operating and sacrificing. Humans don't behave like tortoises. We don't lay our eggs and then walk off, leaving the offspring to fend for themselves. That wouldn't work; they would very quickly die. We birth our babies, and we stay with them, and our community protects and nurtures the children and babies, and this continues throughout the life cycle.

Adults need this system too. We know that being isolated, or lonely, or having problems with interpersonal relationships, or being bullied at work, is bad for our health. Relationships and friendships matter. Both intimate ones, and superficial ones. Just everyday chitchat has been shown to be good for us, lifting our mood and helping us to live longer. Some studies show that relationships are more important for our longevity than healthy eating, regular exercise and quitting smoking. The soothing/affiliative/connected-focused system is about feeling safe in the presence of others, feeling cared for, and caring for others, feeling loved and nurtured, feeling loving and nurturing.

When this soothing/affiliative/connected-focused system is activated, an array of interconnected phenomena plays out. Hormonally, oxytocin and endorphins are released; neurologically, specific areas of the brain become active; physiologically, our heart rate slows and regulates, blood pressure drops, breathing becomes deeper and more regulated; cognitively, our thinking slows down; emotionally, we are more likely to feel relaxed and calm; behaviourally, we are more likely to interact playfully or warmly with others, and generally not do too much that is effortful.

This system is of interest to midwives because it is when this system is activated that childbirth and breastfeeding happen optimally. It is also of interest to psychologists, because it is the key to managing difficult emotions such as anxiety and depression. Research shows that when we learn to activate our soothing/compassionate system, we deactivate the threat system, thereby bringing relief from emotional problems. And it is of interest to immunology because we also know that when we activate the soothing/compassionate system on a regular basis, it has the effect of engaging and boosting our immune system, enhancing our sleep, boosting digestion and maximising our physical and emotional health (Uvnäs-Moberg).

WHAT IS COMPASSION AND HOW IS IT DIFFERENT TO EMPATHY AND SYMPATHY?

Compassion is a function of our care-giving/receiving nature, inbuilt in all of us. We were evolved to care for each other, as a strategy for the survival of our species. Compassion is defined as 'sensitivity to the suffering of others, with a motivation to ease their suffering'. Compassion is not quite the same as sympathy and empathy, but sympathy and empathy are a part of the process. According to Gilbert, we need to be able to be empathic and sympathetic if we are to be compassionate. This is because sympathy is the process of being moved by someone else's suffering. Empathy involves understanding their suffering. We need empathy and sympathy to be caringly sensitive to suffering. But knowing that someone is suffering is not enough – we also have to be *motivated* to do something to help. It might seem to you that empathy, sympathy, and compassion are all the same thing. But they are not, and this has been shown by the remarkable work of Tania Singer and her colleagues. Using brain imaging, they showed us that when people are actively empathic (they are shown pictures of people suffering, and they are asked to really relate to, and understand the suffering of those in the pictures), the stress centres in their brain light up. They become stressed. The threat system gets activated. Conversely, using the same images of people suffering, when those in the brain scanners are asked to be actively compassionate (imagine themselves comforting and helping the sufferers) then they find that completely different parts of the brain light up – those related to the mammalian care-giving system! In other words, the soothing/compassionate system is activated with compassion, but not with empathy. Empathy on its own is draining, exhausting and painful, because we feel their suffering almost as though we feel it ourselves. Compassion is not stressful; it actually feels fine, and can even feel really good. It is the reason that most healthcare professionals enter their profession – they want to connect with people and help people. In order to get a better understanding of this, consider the following scenario. Imagine that you are in a playground, and your child or niece falls over in front of you and grazes her knee badly. She is distraught. You can react with empathy by understanding and feeling her pain. 'Oh my goodness, I remember when that happened to me as a child, the blood is terrifying, the pain is so acute that you think you've been seriously injured, it's so scary, it's just awful'. You would not be much use to the child with empathy and sympathy alone! And you would be quite stressed yourself, so you probably would never work in healthcare! What is needed, is a bit of compassion thrown into the mix. That would look a bit like this: 'Oh you poor thing. That hurts, I know it does. Come here and have a cuddle. Don't you worry about it, it'll be just fine, there there [cuddle, stroke and kiss child]'. And within minutes, you both feel better. Hopefully, you can really sense the difference now, and why those brain scans are so different according to whether the person is exercising their empathy skills alone, or whether they are also being compassionate. What is also interesting about Singer's research is that it demonstrates that compassion can be learned and strengthened. It might be innate, but it is an innate gift which we can hone and build upon.

THE POWER OF COMPASSION FOR HEALING

It is a goal of the NHS to provide compassionate care, and it is enshrined in their policies and (supposedly) procedures. This is because the research is clear; compassionate care helps people to heal. (It also dramatically reduces formal complaints, which, to be fair, may also be a main driver of NHS policies). The soothing/compassionate system is associated with hormones which also enhance basic bodily functioning, such as sleep, digestion, infection control, and the immune system. It has been termed the 'rest and restore' system for this reason (Uvnäs-Moberg). Compassionate care has been shown to benefit patient recovery in many ways, including fewer complications, faster rates of recovery, greater survival rates and earlier discharges from hospital (Youngson). Compassionate care has also been shown to benefit practitioners, and protect them against mental health problems, burnout and suicide attempts (Shanafelt, 2009).

When we tell children who are hurting that we will 'kiss it better', we are actually triggering their healing by activating the soothing/compassionate/rest-and-restore system. When a midwife you trust tells you that she hears you, and she cares about you, and that you are doing an amazing job, your soothing/compassionate system is also triggered, and that helps your labour along. Or, in the case of an emergency, it helps you to stay calm enough to not panic, which could inhibit the work of the doctors, and/or impede your physical and emotional recovery. Compassionate care also helps the midwife, because her job is activating the pleasurable feelings associated with compassionate caring (although she must be given the resources and the autonomy needed, in order to actually be able to help), thereby reducing her chances of burning out emotionally or becoming distant and detached from women in labour.

THE POWER OF ATTENTIVE LISTENING

Compassion is key to midwifery. Midwifery involves being able to be 'with woman' while those that she serves embark on their journey of pregnancy, birth and beyond. During pregnancy, during birth, and after birth, we know that the mother's relaxation levels are important. Michel Odent, the natural birth obstetrician, writes that 'when you meet a pregnant woman, it is your duty to protect her emotional state'. This is because her hormones affect the growing baby. We want the mother to be in the soothing/compassionate system often, so that her body can rest and restore and grow optimally. So that she can have the luxury of thriving, without her mind and body having to prioritise survival by managing threats, fears and concerns. Midwives are a part of this process, helping mums to feel valued and important by listening to them. Listening has many powers that we have yet to fully understand. Lown, the renowned cardiologist, wrote in 1996 about the lost art of healing and the importance of attentive listening.

'it is impossible to treat a patient optimally without the basic 'care' that allows for positive emotions to displace anxiety or hostility, which in turn influence healing processes within limits as is now scientifically understood at the levels of neurology, immunology, and endocrinology'

He also believed that listening to the patient led to more success, in terms of diagnosis as well as treatments – more useful than a myriad of fancy technical equipment. I know about the powers of listening first-hand, because I am a therapist. Compassionate care and listening forms the basis of any good therapy. Research shows us time and time again that the type of therapy is much less important to recovery than the nature of the relationship between the therapist and the client. Being listened to by someone who is motivated and able to help you (someone who is compassionate) is very powerful for healing. I guess it has something to do with the activation of the placebo effect, along with the activation of the soothing/ compassionate system. In the midwifery field, Jennie Joseph, a remarkable midwife who runs a birth centre in Florida, has shown us the power of compassionate care during pregnancy. In her own words:

'We figured out that just being compassionate, open, trusting, listening; those kinds of behaviours, have literally eradicated prematurity in the population of women that I serve, and I do serve the majority of women of colour, women who are at risk for these poor outcomes, suddenly they're thriving'. Joseph, quoted from a BBC Radio 4 interview, 2019.

Prematurity is the leading cause of neonatal death, and having a baby in NICU is a major cause of maternal PTSD, so to be able to eradicate this is a powerful force for health care. Jennie Joseph regards physiological and emotional support as synonymous. Her aims are not to have a live baby and a live mother, but to have a thriving baby and a thriving mother. 'What I'm doing is not even expensive, it's care that's going to keep you safe, the outcomes are clear.' She argues that communicating to a woman that she is welcomed, supported, and that the midwife cares about her as a human being, makes this phenomenal difference to outcome. It makes complete sense to me, and it's exciting that science is beginning to catch up with this intuitive wisdom, by providing us with neuropsychological evidence of why and how that works. The compassionate system in the brain and body releases hormones that activate our healing and wellbeing. This effect is stronger when we feel supported and nurtured by health professionals.

Compassionate midwifery is also important for labour and birth, as well as for pregnancy. In terms of reducing birth trauma, we know that compassionate midwifery serves to reduce the chances of developing PTSD (Ayers et al.). Compassionate care is a health intervention in its own right. When birth attendants listen to women who feel vulnerable, women then feel that the staff have their back, and then you are improving patient safety, reducing risk and increasing the chances of a good outcome. Women know this at an intuitive level – they sense compassionate care when they get it. They know that compassionate care is about the relationship between them and the midwife, and that it is an effective intervention for relieving their suffering (Menage, 2020). For fathers too, compassionate care from the staff is regarded as important. In a study looking at birth trauma among fathers, it was found that fathers value the relationship with the midwives. 'When participants reported that staff were calm and communicated with the couple, this appeared to ease the father and act as a protective factor in their overall view of the experience and how they felt after the birth' (Daniels, 2020).

THE IMPORTANCE OF CONTINUITY OF CARER

In order to activate the soothing/compassionate system in pregnancy and birth, the nature of the relationship matters, and it is much easier to build a relationship if you already know the person. One of the challenges of midwifery is shift changes, or team changes during labour. As a father puts it in one study: 'Unfortunately, the shift changed right before things escalated, so we didn't have much opportunity to build a rapport with the new midwife' (Daniels, 2020). This added to his feelings of trauma after the birth.

Continuity of carer is a form of service delivery that enables the relationship between the midwife and those she serves to thrive. We have known for a long time that having a birth doula in the room reduces the chances of having a caesarean birth, an instrumental birth and postnatal depression, and increases the chances of a shorter labour and satisfaction with the birth (Fukuzawa, 2017). All of those factors are associated with birth trauma. John Kennell famously asserted that 'if a doula were a drug it would be unethical not to use it'.

I have often had the pipe dream that my job as a doula will become redundant when midwives are able to provide what doulas provide: time to develop a relationship, time to care, time to listen, the freedom to use their intuition, the ability to get to know the woman during pregnancy, to be there for her and with her, during and after her labour, available to focus on her emotional wellbeing throughout. That, I understand, is what brings midwives into the profession. It is the inability to do those things that drives compassionate midwives out of the system. It is what midwives and women want. So, let's keep shouting about it. If we enable midwives to provide compassionate care, we improve birth and if we improve birth, we reduce the risk of birth trauma.

COMPASSIONATE CARE BENEFITS THE BABY TOO

Compassionate care is, in my view, key to reducing birth trauma. This needs to be understood at a systemic level, so that it is a factor in the recruitment, training, and retention of staff, so that we are listening to midwives and to women, so that we are valuing and financially rewarding 'soft' skills, so that we are providing work environments and schedules that facilitate compassionate care. This will benefit healthcare professionals, mothers, fathers, and babies. It helps to set up the mother-partner-baby triad in a strong, resilient, loving way.

We know that a good attachment between mother and baby sets the baby up with health benefits that last a lifetime. When the mother feels empowered, proud and safe, she can then look after the health of her baby, creating a nest of safeness and love for the baby. We know that a mentally healthy mother is good for a baby. A system which attends to the emotional wellbeing, as well as the physical needs, of baby, mother and father, may have benefits that last for the rest of that baby's life. For a truly compassionate system, we also need that system to understand that there is no division between mental and physical: they are one and the same.

BREAKING THE MIND-BODY BARRIER

Imagine that you were suffering from severe stomach pain. Imagine that you call an ambulance, and go into hospital for investigations. Imagine that after many scans, blood tests and X-rays, you are told there is nothing physically wrong. Imagine being told that you will be referred to see a psychologist because the pain is 'all in the mind'. How would you feel? Would you believe it? Would you understand it? Would you tell all your friends? Or would you be a little embarrassed?

In our society, there is a basic misunderstanding of the connection between mind and body. We separate it out, as though they are two fairly unrelated entities, only really interested in the physical aspects of the body, while ignoring the less tangible aspects of the mind. Furthermore, there is some shame associated with a phenomenon being psychological, as though that somehow means we are 'making it up' or it 'isn't real – it's just psychological'. Other societies don't share this view. They regard mind and body as part of the whole spirit of a person, something to be addressed in its wholeness, viewing the physical and the emotional as one interactive energy system. As a psychologist, you can imagine how interesting this gets for me!

Nowhere has the mind-body distinction become more problematic than in the field of maternity care. The world of obstetrics and gynaecology is interested in getting the baby out with two people alive by the end of the process. Birth is not viewed as a psychological process, never mind a spiritual process whereby the mind-body is working in a holistic way, transforming two beings such that one can breathe in air through their lungs for the first time, and the other can learn to slow down enough to want to nurture and protect this little being. But birth is very much a psychological process. Science has been telling us this for years. We know that in order to birth without intervention, the mother needs to release the hormone oxytocin, and to release oxytocin, she needs to feel safe. If you get her psychology wrong (her environment, the way she is being treated by others, or even the things she experienced in the past), her hormones won't respond, and she will struggle to birth the baby. Science is finally catching up with what most other societies have known all along – that mind and body cannot be separated. We know that how we choose to breathe affects what happens with our heart, our blood pressure, our immune system, our ability to feel love and be loved, and more. This is because how we breathe affects our central nervous system, and our central nervous system is associated with hormones and emotions, as well as the more physical stuff like our heartbeat and blood pressure. For years, we have known that the mind can heal us physically (the placebo effect) but we have brushed it off as a problem, rather than as clear evidence that something can never be 'all in the mind', or evidence that the mind is a powerful physical force.

THE PLACEBO AND NOCEBO EFFECTS

The placebo effect is the ability of our body to literally heal itself, with the power of expectation and belief that it will do so. In other words, psychological belief and phenomena are intrinsically entwined with real biological phenomena.

Did you know that there is also something called the nocebo effect? That is the ability of our bodies to become ill, through the power of belief. If you believe that the pain of labour will be excruciating, and is dangerous, then you are more likely to feel excruciating pain. This is not open to dispute. It is borne out very clearly in research on pain and the placebo/nocebo effect. We don't yet know how it works, but the impact of language will be a small part of it. Language has a physiological impact on our bodies. For example, if I use words like 'disgust' or 'slime' or 'rotting stench' you will have a biochemical/hormonal reaction to the words. You will also have a behavioural reaction, though you might not notice this. Maybe your face will scrunch up a bit, maybe you'll back off ever so slightly and turn your head to the side, maybe your shoulders will come up. These are all intuitive signs of disgust, and they are associated with the stress system and its related hormones. The nocebo effect might activate the body's stress system, which may interrupt the body's natural healing process, as it enters 'survive' mode rather than 'thrive' mode. Of course, it does more than that, because the nocebo effect creates the *specific* health problem that has been suggested via language. If you are told that a certain pill has the side effect of headache, you are more likely to get a headache, specifically. Brain scans show us that when something is described to us, our brains imagine what is being described (for example, pain) and the parts of the brain that light up are the parts that light up when those things are actually happening to you (the pain centres of your brain!). This throws into dispute something the medical profession does every day – telling patients what the risks and side effects of every procedure might be. In doing so, we are probably causing harm.

The placebo effect, on the other hand, seems to activate something completely different from our stress system. It seems to activate our healing, rest and restore system, which is mediated by oxytocin. If I use the words 'smooth, beautiful, lovely, relaxing, happy' then your hormonal/ biochemical reaction is more likely to be that of oxytocin and endorphins. Your behavioural reaction is more likely to be relaxed shoulders, forehead smoothing out, maybe even a little smile. If those words are used in conjunction with something physiological (such as breastfeeding for example), then, as you imagine 'relaxed breastfeeding', the parts of your brain that are activated while you breastfeed may light up as if you are actually breastfeeding in a relaxed way. When I had my first baby, the two midwives looked at each other and one said to the other 'She has perfect-sized nipples for breastfeeding, doesn't she?' I was a little taken aback by the notion that the size of nipples mattered (it doesn't, by the way) but I then went on to breastfeed my firstborn with absolutely no problems whatsoever (unlike my subsequent two, with whom I had a few more issues). I will never know, but I really do think that the certainty with which those midwives used the words 'perfect' set me up mentally for the best start possible on my breastfeeding journey. The use of language, positivity, encouragement and reassurance may have a very profound impact on our abilities to become pregnant, gestate to full term, birth smoothly and breastfeed successfully. The research so far is beginning to suggest that, but there is so much more to be done to convince the scientific community, and those that want an evidence base for all that we do. But in actuality, maybe all we had to do in the first place was listen to the women we serve. They tell us, time and time again, that support and encouragement matter so much to them. Midwives tell us, time and time again, that they value having time to care, to listen, and to develop meaningful relationships with the families that they serve.

So the emotional and physical can no longer be separated. But we don't even have the language yet to talk about this 'thing' that is both physical and mental. It makes my job as a psychologist quite difficult at times. I know that emotional care literally heals us physically. The placebo effect literally heals us, and we are now beginning to understand the process that is at play. Finally, science is studying how to activate and enhance the placebo effect, rather than merely how to avoid it. And do you know what the most powerful activator of the placebo effect is? It is the relationship between the healer and the healed. If a mother experiences the medic or midwife or practitioner as wise, warm and compassionate, then the effect of the placebo is stronger. Feeling listened to, understood and cared about is important. The research on this is coming out very strongly. It's an exciting time. We are learning that compassion is a powerful force in healing. We are learning that the power of feeling cared for has a dramatic impact on our physical wellbeing. We are learning that being listened to makes people feel heard, and when they feel heard, they stop struggling, and they relax, and they heal. We are also learning that enabling staff to be compassionate in their job reduces the chances of them suffering secondary trauma. Taking care of our midwives, doctors, and midwifery care assistants is key to reducing trauma in both care professionals and in the women, men and babies that they serve.

– 3 –

THE PSYCHOLOGY
OF BIRTH TRAUMA

YOU HAVE TWO BRAINS: YOUR EMOTIONAL BRAIN AND YOUR THINKING BRAIN

Sometimes, our emotional brain and our thinking brain are in disconnect. For example, my thinking brain might *know* logically that a teeny spider can't hurt me. But my emotional brain might still behave as though I am in mortal danger, as I run screaming from the room. The emotional mind and the logical mind are working independently, and this can cause problems.

As humans, we have a brain which works a lot like other mammals. Your mammalian, emotional brain involves feelings such as fear, joy, excitement and affection. It drives behaviour such as loving interaction or aggressive fighting and competitive behaviour. This is our emotional brain, and it is common to all mammals, not just humans. However, we are very different to other mammals (as far as we know!) because as humans, we have a unique thinking and talking ability. Our brains have evolved special skills, housed in the outermost layer of our brain known as the neocortex (or 'new' cortex). These added skills, which we have but other mammals don't, involve our ability to engage in logical, rational thinking, and to talk and plan. For that reason, it has been called the logical brain, or rational brain, or computer brain. Its skills include the ability to plan, daydream, ruminate, worry, fantasise, talk and problem-solve.

Another way of thinking about these skills is to consider that they basically involve the ability to project our experience into the future: 'I'm going on holiday in March, I can't wait to sip a cocktail by the beach, I must remember to sort out my passport, I feel guilty about leaving the dog, I'm super-excited but a little worried', and so on. All these feelings that are running through me, when all I'm doing is sitting at my desk drinking a cup of tea! My imagination is fuelling my experience.

We, as humans, also have the ability to project our experiences back into the past: 'I enjoyed last night, but I don't know what Jane made of it. She seemed a little off. Maybe she's a bit stressed. Maybe I said something that annoyed her. I wish I had asked her'. And we can experience a wonderful mixture of the past and the future in one little second: 'I think Jane was actually not in a good place, and I might have been a little insensitive, so I will go and get a card for her tomorrow, during my lunch break'.

This is an ability that is wonderful for us as humans, but it is also problematic. This is because we can spend a lot of time in a stressful state, while just sitting drinking a cup of tea. Animals don't have this problem. Did you know that if a dog has a nasty fight with another dog, her stress levels will rise at the time of the fight, but within about half an hour, the dog's physiology is back to a normal resting state. Her heart rate has stabilised, and she can relax again. However, if I got into a fight, I know I would not be back to normal after half an hour. The 'new' part of my thinking brain would be going nineteen-to-the-dozen: 'Oh my goodness, I can't believe what just happened, it came out of nowhere, I didn't do anything to provoke it, or did I? No, I didn't, how dare she say that to me, I could have been hurt, what if she had had a knife, where does she live, what if I see her again tomorrow?' and so on. My anxiety about the attack could go on for days and weeks. Sometimes, there's a benefit to being a dog!

This ability to let our minds run away with us, and fuel anxiety, is at the root of a lot of mental health problems. When we have been traumatised, our minds can become 'stuck' in a state of fight or flight, and unable to come back down into a resting state. There are a number of ways to 'manage' the stressful thinking that can dominate our minds at times, and one very powerful way to do it is to practise mindfulness. Take a look at Chapter 4 for psychological tips and techniques for helping your mind to come back down into a more relaxed place.

ARE YOU STRESSED, BUSY OR RELAXED? THE THREE WAYS OF 'BEING'

As mentioned above, it is because we are all human beings that we have the ability to activate feelings of stress involuntarily, just by thinking about particular things that have happened in the past or things that might happen in the future. As we do so, there is a cascade effect, involving hormones, thoughts, feelings and behaviours, in our endocrine system and our brains, activating the 'threat' system in our bodies. I described the threat system in Chapter 2.

This cascade of reactions is all associated with stress. Hormones released include adrenaline and cortisol. Physiologically, you get increased heart rate, irregular shallow breathing, higher blood pressure. Your thinking will change, to be more negative, more catastrophic, more suspicious or more blinkered. Feelings will ensue such as anxiety, anger, or hopelessness, and behaviours will accompany this system, such as wanting to run away, hide or lash out. This can all happen without us really even being aware that it is happening! This threat system is so-called because it is a system which evolved in humans to alert us to danger, and to help us to protect ourselves from danger. It doesn't feel good, but, just like physical pain, it is there for a reason, and that reason is to try to protect us. When we have been traumatised, the threat system has been well and truly switched on. However, unlike other animals, human beings can't switch it off so easily, because our imagination keeps reminding us of what happened. We don't forget about it, and can't go back to eating grass, like a zebra might do only hours after it has been chased by a lion. We stay in the horror of what happened, in our minds, which affects our bodies as if we are still in danger. Even if the event was many years ago.

But here is a question that is worth asking: when our minds and bodies are *not* activating the threat system (or the fight or flight system), what *are* we activating instead? Well, you might remember from Chapter 2 that according to Gilbert's three systems model, there are two other major systems that are associated with being human (and mammalian, for that matter). These are important, because in them, lies the key to recovery. They are the drive system (or busy system), and the soothing/compassionate system (or relaxed system). The drive system is a 'being busy' system, or a motivation system. It is associated with the hormones dopamine and serotonin, with future-orientated thinking, with behaviour that is active, alert, driven, and emotions such as pride, achievement and excitement.

The second system, the soothing/compassionate system, is also known as the relaxation system, or the familial/connection system. This is associated with relaxation and bonding hormones such as oxytocin and endorphins. It is associated with a slowing down of thought, to mere observation or a trance-like state. Physiologically, it is accompanied by a regular, slower heart rate, belly breathing and reduced blood pressure. Behaviourally, the soothing system is deactivating – it slows us down, makes us less inclined to get up, and more inclined to just rest. It is that Sunday afternoon on the sofa feeling, or resting in the sun on holiday. It feels nice, so we tend to want to stay in it. While in it, our bodies go about resting and restoring, and building our immune system, which is why it has also been termed the 'rest and digest' or the 'calm and connect' system (Kerstin Uvnäs-Moberg). As well as having health-giving aspects such as enhanced sleep, digestion and immune system, it is also associated with affection, touch, birth, breastfeeding, bonding with your baby, and healing from trauma. You can see why I outline the soothing system and its functions for you! The point is that we can learn to activate, or switch on, each of these systems, according to our will. It is going to be your means of getting better, of healing from a bad birth. Learning to reactivate this system is going to boost your recovery.

We will be returning to the concept of these three systems later in the book. For the time being, suffice it to say that during your birth, if you ended up traumatised, the chances are that you were not experiencing the soothing system in action. You did not feel protected, safe, cared for or soothed. As we outlined in the first chapter, birth is biologically designed to happen while we feel safe, awash with oxytocin and endorphins, and when it doesn't, it can cause problems for our psyche. It is more likely that, during your birth, or while you were trying to breastfeed, you were in the threat system, feeling unsafe, unprotected and flooded with adrenaline and cortisol.

Having said that, birth trauma isn't only about how you were at the time of the event, it is about how you recover from that awful event. It is about how you are *now*. When we are traumatised, the brain's threat system carries on being overactive, after the scary event has passed. It is kicking off randomly, when it doesn't need to, or when you least expect it to. It is stuck in the threat system, unable to feel relaxed and safe. Because you can't get into the soothing system (which is also your healing and recovery system), your mind and body struggle to heal naturally. In order for you to recover, we need your brain to get out of the threat system, and into the soothing system. Once you are able to feel safe again, to relax again, then your mind and body will start to heal naturally. In Chapter 4, you will be guided through different strategies and tips for achieving this.

THE FACTS: WHAT CAUSES BIRTH TRAUMA?

Trigger warning: contains reference to traumatic births and obstetric violence.

What causes birth trauma? This is a million-dollar question that I wish I had the answer to! As with many things that involve people, psychology, sociology and culture, the answer is multi-faceted. There are many theories and findings out there. It has always been commonplace to look for reasons why the woman was vulnerable in the first place (what we call predisposing factors) – for example, research has shown that women with a previous history of mental health problems are more likely to experience birth trauma.

We also know that women who have experienced sexual abuse in the past are more likely to be traumatised. Women who had a fear of birth beforehand and women who had complications during pregnancy are also more at risk, statistically speaking. Women who have previously suffered from PTSD are also more at risk. (This is statistical by the way – it doesn't mean that *you* are *likely* to be traumatised if you've been abused in the past, it means that you are slightly *more* likely than someone who hasn't survived previous abuse.) There is plenty of research that has managed to identify pre-disposing factors.

However, I'm not a great fan of this approach, because I

think it focuses our attention on the woman, as though she is the one at fault. And by doing that, it draws us away from the real problem. The problem is not in the woman. The problem lies with the system. For example, what is it about our maternity system that makes women who have been previously sexually assaulted more vulnerable to developing PTSD? That is an important question that needs answering. I'll ask it again.

WHY IS IT THAT HAVING A BABY CAN RE-TRIGGER OLD MEMORIES OF SEXUAL ASSAULT?

Is it something about the maternity system? If so, we need to know that, in order to put it right. It really isn't rocket science, to understand that the maternity system can open up previous traumatic memories of sexual abuse. For a start, it often takes the power away from the women and puts it in the hands of the doctors. For example, the 'routine' practice of internal examinations (or, rather, having fingers put into your vagina), being put on your back, having medics lean over you, being told you're a 'good girl', having more than one person stare at your vagina without addressing you, being told to stay still and so on, being told to leave your dignity at the door, to not question those in authority, all sounds pretty unappealing.

As I say, it seems obvious that such 'routine' practices within midwifery might ignite previous memories of abuse. These practices are institutionalised and normalised. I work with women, midwives and men who are amazed when I tell them that it is possible to have a baby without internal examinations. That, in itself blows my mind. Why would anyone think that you can't have a baby without an internal exam? You can have a baby much more easily without someone shoving their fingers up to your cervix. Babies have been born without medical or digital intervention for millions of years. And yet, internal exams are done routinely, and sometimes hourly for women who are in labour. It is done in order to 'measure progress', so that we can see how opened her cervix is.

Imagine if I wanted to make sure that a person was able to empty their bladder to avoid infection, and I did so by watching them, and poking at their bladder every few minutes to see how 'full' it is, and then said they were failing when their body couldn't let go enough just to have a wee. It's a crazy way to behave. It's a risky way to behave if you are hoping to avoid psychological fall-out and distress. And yet, it is seen not only as normal, but also as necessary, in order to have a baby. And when women come away traumatised from it, we blame them for having 'predisposing factors'.

It doesn't have to be that way. I have been at many births where the midwives have not done a single internal exam because the birthing mother didn't want them to. And that was respected. And do you know what? The baby was born. I know of doctors who get on their hands and knees to assist a birth with a ventouse suction, so that the woman doesn't have to get on her back. When women who have been traumatised were asked what care providers could have done to prevent the trauma, they said: communicated better with me, listened to me more, supported me more, practically and emotionally (Hollander et al).

I have worked with many women (especially survivors of abuse) who love the birth pool, because 'no one can touch me (or assault me) in a birth pool, and I stay in control of what is on show'. And yet, birth pools are still so difficult to access in many maternity services, on account of a myriad of bizarre excuses and problems. Our society sometimes presumes that birth trauma exists because the nature of birth is inherently traumatic. I disagree. I actually like the term 'obstetric trauma' rather than birth trauma, because I do believe that a great deal of birth trauma is caused by a system which is damaging. Oftentimes, it isn't the nature of birth itself that is traumatising. Birth can actually be quite empowering and wonderful for the mother.

OTHER CAUSES OF BIRTH TRAUMA

Let's take a look at what the research is telling us about the causes of birth trauma. Susan Ayers and her team have researched this extensively and come up with some interesting findings. There seem to be two important areas of interest. One is, predictably, the level of obstetric intervention, complication and urgency, and whether or not your baby ended up in special care. If you have an operative delivery (forceps or caesarean section), or your baby had complications, then you are more at risk of developing birth trauma. It might be worth mentioning at this point though, that statistics are based on very large numbers of people, so they actually tell us very little about your individual situation.

For example, statistics tell us that the average height for women is 162cm, but that doesn't help me know how tall I am. Statistics might tell us that being tall makes you more likely to bump your head, but that doesn't mean that I am at risk of bumping my head. Nor does it mean that if I do bump my head, it was because I am tall. (It might have been for any number of reasons, such as I've had a drink, or I left something lying around in my bedroom, or I was trying to avoid someone, or I've got a brain tumour and so on.) My point is this. Just because you had an operative delivery, does not mean you are *likely* to get birth trauma. In fact, it cannot predict anything for you. It just says the chances are slightly (very slightly – almost negligibly in individual cases) higher.

The second factor which seems to increase the risk of developing PTSD after childbirth is, according to Ayers's research, perceived lack of interpersonal care and support during the birth. This is in line with my personal experience of working with women who have been traumatised by their birth. They did not feel safe or supported by the midwives or doctors. They did not feel listened to. They feel that control was taken from them.

According to the research, the lack of support is more important than the obstetric interventions. Furthermore, when a woman *does* feel supported, this reduces the risk of trauma caused by obstetric intervention. In Ayers's words 'support that women receive during birth is absolutely critical, it can buffer against the negative consequences of a stressful birth'. Furthermore, Ayers writes, 'unlike many other postpartum psychological problems, there is the potential to prevent postpartum PTSD by changing maternity care to reduce the number of women who experience birth as traumatic'. The presence of a birth doula (who you get to know during your pregnancy and who stays with you throughout the labour), has long been shown to reduce the risk of all kinds of obstetric interventions. We now know that continuous support during labour from midwives is important too (Bohren et al, 2017).

One of the most immediately effective ways of changing maternity care is to provide continuity of carer. This means that the woman in labour has birth attendants whom she already knows. Someone she met during her pregnancy. Not a stranger. This makes sense to me, psychologically speaking, because we are evolved to have some reticence and hesitation when meeting strangers – especially when we need to put our lives (and the life of our baby) in their hands. It's so much easier if we've met them before. Also, arguably, a woman is more likely to be listened to and taken seriously if the staff know her already.

Continuity of carer has many proven benefits, including reduced rates of episiotomy or instrumental birth, reduced rates of preterm birth, reduced rates of miscarriage and neonatal death, and women reporting more satisfaction with various aspects of their care (Cochrane systematic review, 2016). It's a no-brainer. It would also save money, because it would reduce intervention during the birth itself, and it would reduce PTSD rates after the birth. It is kinder. I don't know why it doesn't happen. I don't know why maternity services continually disband services that offer it. Sometimes I feel that it is because it involves strong midwives being strong for birthing women in order to make those women even stronger. Sometimes I feel that it is patriarchy keeping hold of the control, and maintaining a system whereby we break midwives and mothers, thereby keeping them weaker and quieter.

WE SHOULD RENAME IT OBSTETRIC TRAUMA, NOT BIRTH TRAUMA

It has taken some time for birth trauma to be recognised as a real thing. People used to think that PTSD happened after horrific experiences like being in a war zone, not during a normal process like birth. In order to understand it, some people conclude that birth trauma happens because birth is, in itself, a horrible, painful ordeal. I'm not one who agrees with this. That's a bit like saying that rape trauma happens because sex is, in itself, a horrible, painful ordeal. Not true. The sex isn't the problem; it's the circumstances around the sex that lead us to call it traumatic. The power relationship, the lack of consent, the circumstances, the aggression, and more, make it rape. I think it is the same with birth trauma, and I would like to see a recognition that it isn't birth that is traumatic *per se*. It is the circumstances around it that make it so. For that reason, I think the term obstetric trauma is more appropriate.

PSYCHOLOGICAL TRAUMA ISN'T EVEN ABOUT WHAT HAPPENED

If you are questioning whether or not you have been traumatised by your birth, remember that 'feeling that the birth was horrible or traumatic' is indicative of possible trauma. This is (almost) enough. You don't need to have had a dramatic emergency during the birth. Psychological trauma isn't about what actually happened: it's about the psychological injury, or the aftermath, of what happened.

I've heard some birth stories that are so horrible, my insides shrink when I hear them. But the mums are fine with it. I hear other birth stories that sound like good, straightforward births on paper. But the mums are sobbing with grief and horror while they tell me. How can that be?

Well, trauma is about the *injury*, not the event. It's like breaking a bone. I might fall down a big flight of stairs, and walk away unscathed. On the other hand, I might trip up over nothing, and break my ankle. You cannot predict this, or control it. The person who broke their ankle is not weaker or more stupid, and they cannot 'pull themselves together'. They just got injured. Birth trauma is the same. Yes, you are more likely to break your ankle falling from a great height, and you are more likely to be traumatised during an emergency procedure, but sometimes we break our ankle tripping over a kerb, and sometimes we get birth trauma because we weren't listened to. So, as a psychologist, when assessing for trauma, I'm way more interested in how the person feels about the birth, than what actually happened at the birth.

HOW IS ALL THIS SUPPOSED TO HELP YOU?

When you know that the reasons that you suffer are not to do with you having failed in some way, and when you know that your feelings are valid, then that is the first step to letting go of any self-blame, and being able to acknowledge your feelings. These are important steps to recovery, and ones which I always address during therapy. You are not to blame for feeling this way. Your feelings are a result of what happened to you. Your feelings are valid, and they matter.

IS IT PTSD OR NOT? DIAGNOSTIC CRITERIA AND THE DIFFERENCE BETWEEN A BAD BIRTH AND POST-TRAUMATIC STRESS DISORDER

Psychiatry is a funny old business. It is interested in mental illnesses, and in particular, it wants to know how to diagnose them so that they can be treated. It is a disease and medical model in action. Professionals, researchers, practitioners and academics look for patterns in people who are struggling, gather them together, name them, and then publish them in a doctor's 'diagnostic manual' such as the Diagnostic and Statistical Manual of mental disorders (DSM), or the International Classification of Diseases (ICD). While it is trying to copy a medical model, it's not as easy to do this with mental health as it is for some other diseases, because there isn't a 'disease' we can find, like cancer cells or diabetes or blood disorders. There isn't even brain chemistry to see, despite what many pharmaceutical companies would have you believe.

In other words, a lot of psychiatric syndromes are kind of made up, following years of careful observation and analysis. The diagnostic categories are updated every three decades or so, because psychological symptoms change as societies change. For example, not so long ago homosexuality was viewed as a mental disorder. Before that, nymphomania was a psychiatric condition exclusively attributed to women. Nowadays, 'female sexual interest/arousal disorder' is an official category of mental health problems, and is the polar opposite of nymphomania, which says more about our society than it does about mental disorder.

Post-traumatic stress disorder and trauma symptoms are the same. These are psychiatric concepts, and as such, there isn't anything we can 'see' in order to diagnose them. Specialists spend time observing and allocating what they see, they then write down specific 'criteria' that need to be happening, before it can be said that a person is showing signs of a specific problem. We have been doing this with trauma ever since the First World War, when we were faced with cases of what we called 'shell shock' in war veterans. This was the start of our journey into trying to understand trauma: what happens, why it happens, who it happens to, what happens in the brain. PTSD as a syndrome was first introduced as a psychiatric condition in 1980, and it has been through some significant changes since then. Most of these changes have involved a broadening of the concept of trauma, from there just being either PTSD or no PTSD, to a more sophisticated understanding of trauma, which includes other diagnostic categories associated with trauma, such as acute stress reaction and adjustment disorder and the fact that it's not necessarily the event itself that traumatises us, but how we interpret the event, that makes the difference.

Having diagnostic criteria can be helpful, in that it can give a name to your suffering. There are four important aspects that all need to be present for any formal diagnosis of post-traumatic stress disorder.

1 AN EVENT IN WHICH YOU THOUGHT YOU OR SOMEONE ELSE WAS GOING TO DIE/BE HARMED

Firstly, there has to have been an event to speak of. Watching something on television isn't thought to be able to traumatise you, although I think this will change in the near future. Watching something awful happen to someone else counts. So your birthing companion or your midwife could get PTSD from watching your birth, even though he or she wasn't the source of the danger. Maybe your 'event' was a series of events, such as trying to breastfeed over a number of days or weeks. It might feel like it isn't one specific memory, but often people can isolate the event in the form of a few particular images, or 'snippets', or 'hot memories' that epitomise trauma associated with that. According to

Susan Ayers, one in five women, or 20% of women who have had a baby, meet this first criterion. They experience a birth in which they thought that they, or their baby, were going to die or be harmed. That is way too many in my opinion, and begs the question – what is going on in our society and our maternity system to create that much fear?

2 SOME FORM OF ANXIETY OR RELIVING OF THE DISTRESS

Secondly, there has to be some sort of reliving, or anxiety, or distress associated with the memory of the event. This can include flashbacks, or nightmares, or constantly thinking about it when you don't want to, or feeling distressed or anxious every time you are reminded of it. This has to be happening three months or more beyond the date of the traumatising event. You might think that reliving is enough to diagnose PTSD, but it isn't. This is because it is normal to get some reliving and distress after a horrible experience. It is only considered a problem when it lasts for more than three months after the event, and if we are actively pushing it away mentally, on a regular basis. Which takes us to the third criterion: avoidance.

3 YOU AVOID SITUATIONS OR THOUGHTS THAT REMIND YOU OF THE EVENT

Thirdly, avoidance. This takes the form of avoiding anything that reminds you of the traumatising events, such as mother and baby groups, or programmes on television, or conversations about birth, or friends who are pregnant or breastfeeding, and so on. You can also avoid things in your own head – so as soon as the memory surfaces, you develop sophisticated ways to distract yourself or to think about something else, or push it away. Avoidance is an important facet of PTSD, because it is believed that it is avoidance that creates a vicious cycle, in that the brain needs to process the memory, in the form of talking it through, or crying, or thinking about it, but it isn't able to do so because the avoidance strategies are preventing that from happening. This is not voluntary, it is not anyone's fault: it is the brain trying to protect itself from horror.

4 THE EVENT HAS LEFT ITS MARK ON YOUR LIFE, YOUR THOUGHTS OR YOUR BELIEFS

Fourthly, the event has to have had an impact on your general feelings about life and your views about yourself or others. For example, it may have changed how you feel about yourself: you may feel guilty or flawed. It may have changed how you feel about others, or about the NHS, if you feel angry, or it may have led you to feel low in mood because the world doesn't feel like a good place to be.

If you are interested in the full diagnostic criteria, you can find them in the appendices at the end of the book. The diagnostic criteria are useful for research purposes, so that researchers can categorise exactly who they are studying, but I'm not sure how useful they are to you. This is because you may not meet the full criteria for PTSD, but you might be suffering an awful lot with symptoms of trauma nonetheless. Full-blown PTSD is the tip of the iceberg in terms of severity. It affects between 2 and 5% of women who have had babies. However, a much larger group of women have what I would refer to as sub-clinical trauma symptoms. They might not meet the full criteria, but they are suffering, and their feelings matter. So I have created my own list of things that I think are important when women ask me if I think that they have been traumatised. When assessing for trauma, I look (or listen) out for three main things. Having checked that the event happened more than a month ago, I move onto the following clues:

1 IS THE FEELING STILL RAW?

I check whether the person can tell me the story without becoming very upset. When we have lived through a distressing experience, the adage that 'time heals' is often true, but only if we haven't been traumatised. As time moves on, we tend to find that the emotion becomes less raw, and the feelings diminish, even if we still remember exactly what happened. Memory and feelings become disassociated, in that we might still remember the detail of what happened, but the feelings belong in the past. They do not swamp us in the present. This is normal. But not so for trauma. If the experience has left a traumatic imprint, you will find that the feelings do not abate with time. You will find that thinking about it, or talking about it, brings back the feelings as strongly as ever. That is why I ask myself 'Can she tell me what happened without becoming very upset?' If the answer is no, the chances are that the memory has become traumatic for you.

2 DOES IT FEEL LIKE IT ONLY HAPPENED YESTERDAY?

Does the memory *feel* as though it only happened recently, even when it happened months or years ago? In other words, is the memory at the forefront of their minds, rather than a distant memory. If you have been traumatised, the chances are that it will *feel* like it happened recently, even though you *know* it happened a long time ago.

3 ARE YOU STRUGGLING TO MOVE ON FROM IT?

Does the birth play over and over in your mind, and you find that you can't let it go? It's as though it is haunting you, hassling you, constantly there in some way, and preventing you from getting on with your life. Do you want to be able to put it into the past, where you feel it belongs, but you just can't seem to do it?

When I am listening to a birth story, I don't always need to know about the event. I need to know about the reaction to the event. I want to know 'Can you talk about it without crying?' I want to know 'Does it impact on your dreams?' I want to know 'Do you try to shove it to the back of your mind, but you find it impossible?' I want to know 'What impact is it having on your life now?' I also want to know when the birth was. If it was less than four weeks ago, I advise self-care. If it was more than that, I advise treatment for trauma.

It's worth noting that the trauma associated with a memory can be buried successfully for years, only to come back when reminders of it come into your life. You may have got on with life after a difficult experience, only to find it all coming flooding back. In my experience, the most common trigger is getting pregnant again. Suddenly, the previous birth comes to the forefront of your mind, and you find that you can't stop thinking about it, or worrying about it. Or maybe you had to go back into the same hospital, for something unassociated with pregnancy, but being there opened up the feelings again. Or a friend of yours, or even your own daughter, is having a baby. I worked with one woman who had been traumatised 38 years previously, and came to me for help because her daughter was now pregnant. The point is that you may have managed to bury the feelings and get on with life, but the wounds can unfortunately be reopened. And they feel the same. The feelings are raw, it feels recent, and you're struggling to move on from it.

IS IT TRAUMA, OR IS IT DEPRESSION?

One of the problems with identifying whether problems are due to trauma or something else, is that the experiences can be very similar to other problems, such as depression or anxiety. For example, you may find yourself crying a lot, or feeling like you've failed, or have trouble sleeping, or getting angry and irritable with others, or being distracted easily and unable to focus. I have worked with many women who have suicidal thoughts associated with birth trauma. These are all symptoms of depression too. This is why birth trauma is so often missed – professionals miss it too. And to add to the confusion, it could also be the case that you are experiencing both trauma and depression at the same time. What began as birth trauma, can, over time, go on to cause depression, as you struggle to cope with being a mum at the same time as having trauma symptoms.

THE CITY BIRTH TRAUMA SCALE (CITY BITS) FOR ASSESSING BIRTH TRAUMA

Professor Susan Ayers and her team at City Hospital, London, have developed a checklist to help us to assess to what extent you might be suffering from birth trauma. They have developed a robust questionnaire for helping people to explore whether or not they might meet the criteria for a diagnosis of PTSD. It is the first of its kind, because it specifically focuses on birth, and it is welcome. It is printed here so that you can take a look and see that the questions are related to the diagnostic criteria listed above. But you can also have a go at filling it out for yourself if you so choose.

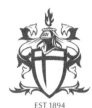

EST 1894

CITY UNIVERSITY LONDON
Birth Trauma Scale

This questionnaire asks about your experience during the birth of your most recent baby. It asks about potential traumatic events during (or immediately after) the labour and birth, and whether you are experiencing symptoms that are reported by some women after birth. Please tick the responses closest to your experience.

What date was your baby born? _____

During the labour, birth and immediately afterwards:		
Did you believe you or your baby would be seriously injured?	Yes	No
Did you believe you or your baby would die?	Yes	No

The next questions ask about symptoms that you might have experienced. Please indicate how often you have experienced the following symptoms in the last week:

Symptoms about the birth*	NOT AT ALL	ONCE	2 - 4 TIMES	5 OR MORE TIMES
Recurrent unwanted memories of the birth (or parts of the birth) that you can't control				
Bad dreams or nightmares about the birth (or related to the birth)				
Flashbacks to the birth and/or reliving the experience				
Getting upset when reminded of the birth				
Feeling tense or anxious when reminded of the birth				
Trying to avoid thinking about the birth				
Trying to avoid things that remind me of the birth (e.g. people, places, TV programs)				
Not able to remember details of the birth				
Blaming myself or others for what happened during the birth				
Feeling strong negative emotions about the birth (e.g. fear, anger, shame)				

* Although these questions refer to the birth, many women have symptoms about events that happened just before or after birth. If this is the case for you, and the events were related to pregnancy, birth or the baby then please answer for these events.

Symptoms that began or got worse since the birth	NOT AT ALL	ONCE	2 - 4 TIMES	5 OR MORE TIMES
Feeling negative about myself or thinking something awful will happen				
Lost interest in activities that were important to me				
Feeling detached from other people				
Not able to feel positive emotions (e.g. happy, excited)				
Feeling irritable or aggressive				
Feeling self-destructive or acting recklessly				
Feeling tense and on edge				
Feeling jumpy or easily startled				
Problems concentrating				
Not sleeping well because of things that are not due to the baby's sleep pattern				
Feeling detached or as if you are in a dream				
Feeling things are distorted or not real				

If you have any of these symptoms:

When did these symptoms start?	
Before the birth	
In the first 6 months after birth	
More than 6 months after birth	
Not applicable (I have no symptoms)	

How long have these symptoms lasted?	
Less than 1 month	
1 to 3 months	
3 months or more	
Not applicable (I have no symptoms)	

Do these symptoms cause you a lot of distress?	Yes	No	Sometimes
Do they prevent you doing things you usually do (e.g. socialising, daily activities)?	Yes	No	Sometimes
Could any of these symptoms be due to medication, alcohol, drugs, or physical illness?	Yes	No	Maybe

Thank you for completing this questionnaire

'City Birth Trauma Scale' questionnaire Version 2.0
© Ayers, Wright and Thornton 2018. Reproduced by kind permission.

THE NEUROLOGICAL BIT: WHAT HAPPENS IN THE BRAIN WHEN A MEMORY BECOMES TRAUMATIC

Psychology is very exciting at the moment in terms of understanding how the brain works. Previously, for thousands of years, the only method we had for understanding what happens in the brain was to remove the brain and take a good look at it after the person had died. Fast-forward to the 21st century, and we begin to see a lot more, thanks to the use of X-rays, CT scans and MRI scans, enabling us to look at the brain while a person is still alive. In terms of neurology, the most exciting advance is the most recent one (developed in the 1990s): functional Magnetic Resonance Imaging (fMRI). An fMRI helps us look at changes in the brain while it is actually working. It's like the difference between a static photo, and a video of the brain in action. This is leading to an explosion in rich discoveries and information about the functioning of the brain, including information about what happens in the brain when we are traumatised. It is a very complex area, but luckily, plenty of helpful psychologists have created simplified versions of what seems to be happening in the brain when we are faced with a flood of overwhelming fear or anxiety. I'm going to try to explain it for you.

There are three areas of the brain that are involved. The first is the amygdala, which is housed deep within the brain. We will call this the 'emotional brain' because it is where most of our basic emotions are housed. The amygdala is responsible for 'spotting' and 'reacting to' danger very quickly. It spots danger based on a combination of instinct and previous experiences. For example, the amygdala is more likely to respond to spiders than it is to a can of beans. And it is more likely to respond to spiders if it has been bitten by one, or has seen someone else be frightened of them. The second area of the brain which seems to be involved in processing trauma is the hippocampus. This area is also in the emotional part of the brain, and is involved in sorting out our memories, particularly in putting memories into historical or long-term memory. We will call this the 'gateway'. The third area of the brain that we are interested in is the neocortex. This is the area that is 'newest' in evolutionary terms, and is responsible for our higher evolved processes such as thinking, planning, talking, logical reasoning and so on. We will call this the 'rational' part of our brain.

The current understanding of what happens during an overwhelmingly threatening situation, is that these three parts of the brain react to danger in the following manner: the amygdala spots the danger, and releases a flood of danger hormones. These danger hormones serve to get the person to act quickly to get themselves safe again. In order to facilitate this, it actively shuts down the ability to think or reason or apply logic, via the hippocampus. This makes sense, because when we are faced with danger, we should not be thinking 'I wonder how dangerous this is, I wonder if it would be better for me to say something, or whether I should just punch someone?' By then, you may have been punched first. So the brain shuts down your ability to think, so that you just react. It's a 'better safe than sorry' mechanism. If it *is* a dangerous situation, you engage your defences. If it turns out not to be a dangerous situation, your thinking comes back on line. It's why I still 'jump' when I hear my cat come in through the cat flap. *After* I have jumped, my thinking brain kicks in with 'Oh, it's just the cat'. To my frustration, it happens every time. Every single time. You would think my brain would learn. But no, it prefers to stay better safe than sorry, in case, next time, it actually is an axe-wielding burglar. So, using the cat example, it goes a bit like this:

1　Amygdala spots danger (noise by door)
2　Hippocampus shuts down thinking (jump out of my skin)
3　Act until danger is over (eyes wide, rush of adrenaline, head spins round to see)

4 Danger is over
5 Then hippocampus activates thinking (it's the cat)
6 Communication happens between the neocortex and the amygdala to rationalise what happened (why do I always let that happen, no worries, I'll go back to watching TV).

In the case of birth, the example might go like this:

1 Amygdala spots danger (I am not being listened to, I don't feel safe)
2 Hippocampus shuts down (freeze)
3 Act until danger is over (numb, unable to react, say nothing)
4 Danger is over
5 The hippocampus activates thinking (I'm going to be okay)
6 Communication happens between the neocortex and the amygdala to rationalise what happened (I got scared there but I'm okay now, and it's over)

When trauma happens, the theory is that the brain gets stuck in a loop, at step 3. The brain fails to realise that the danger is over, because it is playing 'better safe than sorry' and is being flooded with stress hormones that are stopping the brain from 'thinking' and realising that there is no more danger. So it looks more like this:

1 Amygdala spots danger (I am not being listened to)
2 Hippocampus shuts down (freeze)
3 Act until danger is over (numb, unable to react, say nothing)
1 Amygdala spots danger
2 Hippocampus shuts down
3 Act until danger is over
1 Amygdala spots danger
2 And so on…

There's never a chance for the brain to think 'Oh, it's okay now, I can rationalise what happened because I am safe'. When we are stuck in trauma, the brain stays flooded with stress hormones. We stay hyper alert, vigilant, feeling unsafe, jumpy, nervous, stressed, unable to sleep, and the memory keeps playing as though it happened only yesterday, as though it is still raw and real. We might know logically that 'I have a healthy baby and I'm going to be okay', but the amygdala isn't interested in logic (because there is blocked communication between the emotional and the rational parts of the brain. The gateway is stopping the emotional and the rational parts of our brain from communicating). Ruth's experience during therapy is a great illustration of this.

RUTH'S STORY

Ruth came to me for help with birth trauma. The birth had left her with feelings that many mothers will feel familiar with after a difficult and medicalised birth. She felt that she had been not listened to, she had lost control, it was partly her fault, and she felt as if she had been assaulted by the staff. The anger and the horror that she felt were directed at herself to some extent, and at the staff to a larger extent. During therapy, Ruth began to feel listened to. She learnt grounding techniques to help her cope with flashbacks and triggers. As the trauma symptoms lifted, she told me that learning to be calmer had helped her to see what she could not see before. She literally could see stuff she couldn't 'see' before, because she was able to look at her notes for the first time since the birth. (This was not possible before then, because of the severe anxiety and trauma symptoms.) And when she read them, she 'saw' things she hadn't seen before, in terms of her understanding. Although she had been told on numerous occasions that her birth had been a medical emergency, she had not been able to hear that, because the anger was so raw and the distress was so deep.

However, once the trauma symptoms started to lift, she

began to see it differently. She began to feel that the staff were just doing their best. Yes, they made some mistakes, and their communication was left wanting. But 'We all try our best, don't we? We don't all always get it right, do we?' This generous view was more in line with Ruth's premorbid personality. She was generally quite a forgiving, rational, understanding person. That person had temporarily vanished with the trauma, and she had been angry and irrational and awful to live with (her words). Now that her brain was calmer and the symptoms were lifting, she began to feel that the staff had, indeed, been trying to save her life, rather than trying to assault her.

She was still angry and hurt that it had happened. She still felt it was unfair. But she could see that they were in a rush to save her, and that they had tried. That is something she had not been able to see before. Ruth also began to see that far from failing, her body had been incredible to survive the assault/birth, and had managed very successfully to establish a great bond with her son in spite of the rough start that they both had.

WHY HOW YOUR CARE PROVIDERS TREATED YOU CAN BE SO IMPORTANT IN BIRTH TRAUMA

Some people question why the rates of trauma are so high after birth. We have known that trauma is often associated with witnessing a near-death, or something horrific. This makes sense on the battlefield. But in the birthing field? As mentioned earlier in this chapter, with birth, what seems to make a difference is the relationship between the woman who is labouring and her care providers. Why is this? Well, I think it has something to do with the way that we respond to threat.

You are probably already aware of the 'fight or flight' response to danger. The fight/flight option involves an automatic instinct to shout/scream/run when we feel some form of threat or danger. It is activating, and we feel scared, our heart rate goes up, we want to escape, our breathing changes, we feel hot and bothered, and so on. However, there is a catch. This fight or flight response relies on us being stronger, faster, or scarier than the threat. The fight or flight response relies on us being able to *save ourselves*. That's all well and good if you're fit, healthy and strong. But what if you are quite small? Or quite feminine? Or heavily pregnant? Or in the middle of labour? Then the fight or flight response is next to useless. You might be the kind of person who sticks up for yourself, who takes no nonsense, who is confident and assertive. But you might find that when you were in labour, all that went out of the window. Because when women are in labour, and they begin to feel unsafe, then they turn to another form of self-protection. You did not 'fail' to speak up because you are weak, or did anything wrong. It's much more likely that your brain and body switched to another mode of survival, unconsciously and automatically. There are two other options that your brain might have taken.

1 'TEND AND BEFRIEND' RESPONSE TO DANGER

As well as the fight/flight system for survival, humans have developed more sophisticated additional ways of dealing with danger, some of which include social elements of our wiring. We have a network of nerves in the autonomic nervous system that activate a 'social engagement system', whereby we look to others for support and protection. This has been termed the 'tend and befriend' system. The theory is that if we are in danger, we look to other people to provide safety for us, other people who have our back, and who will protect us and stand up for us. Thus, men are more likely to fight or flee their way out of trouble. Childbearing women are arguably more likely to cry for help or stick with people that they trust or feel safe with. If that were the case, then we would expect a *birthing* mother to absolutely use the tend and befriend system to stay safe. It's not much good trying to run or fight when you are in labour. This means that a woman in labour wants to know that those around her have her back. The last thing she will do is annoy, irritate or go against those around her, because she is relying on them to be her support. She needs to know that they will protect her *to the death* if something happens, so she remains as pleasant and agreeable as possible, even when this is completely out of character for her. (Take note: this is not a conscious thing. It's about as automatic as blinking when you hear a loud noise. Your brain does it automatically.)

Let's imagine that the mother is sweet and kind and smiley and begs not to be on her back because she is in a lot of pain, and she gets no response. Or the midwife doesn't seem to be interested. What then? Does it matter? Well, yes. Because it suggests to her that the one person who can keep her and her baby safe doesn't really care! The mother needs to feel that the midwife will protect her. She needs to feel safe. And she doesn't. She feels alone, frightened and unsupported. At her most vulnerable time, when her fight or flight response is inactivated. The brain registers this. Activation of the 'tend and befriend' system is not working. Her brain will then default to the next level of protection – immobilisation, the freeze response.

2 FREEZE RESPONSE

Polyvagal theory suggests that when we are faced with danger that cannot be dealt with by the help of others or by our own efforts, then the body goes into shut-down mode. This is not within our conscious control. It is a defence mechanism so old, that all mammals and reptiles on the planet use it. It comes in the form of feeling unable to move or talk (paralysed) or feeling numb or distanced from the experience (dissociation). Activation of this type of defence mechanism suggests high levels of fear/entrapment, and is associated with the development of PTSD. It partly explains why, even though you might be a very assertive woman in other areas of your life, you didn't assert yourself at the birth of your baby. Your in-built, evolved self-defence mechanism kicked in and you froze, in order to save your or your baby's skin. I often hear women say 'I should have been more assertive', or 'I don't know why I didn't say something' or 'Why didn't I just tell them to stop belittling me' and so on. I'm going to spend a little time on this, because it is common, and very important. The reason it is important is because what is behind the confusion is usually a sense of 'It's my fault. I should have done something different'. If there is one thing that I want this book to communicate, it's that a bad birth is *never your fault*. It's a feeling that Stacey was left with for years, after the birth of her baby.

STACEY'S STORY: 'I WAS ANGRY WITH MYSELF FOR NOT SAYING NO'

Stacey came to me for help with her previous experience of birth trauma with her eight-year-old daughter. Stacey is a very insightful, thoughtful, loving mother, and there was an air of sadness about the 'lost' years. This time was 'lost' in terms of not really knowing how to address what had happened, and also in the sense that her dreams for a carefree babyhood with her daughter had been taken from her.

When Stacey told me about her traumatic birth with her first baby, her story was different to others that I had heard before. At first. I was bamboozled initially by the fact that she had a specific condition which was undiagnosed at the time of the birth. As a result of this, she had to deal with issues which no mother or family should have to face, such as being in and out of hospital for many weeks, being scared for her own life, having to inform medics about her own condition and so on. However, when Stacey elaborated on her birth story, I realised that the narrative was all too familiar to me. I had heard it before, many times, over and over. She told me, in her second session, that she had 'been treated pretty badly' in that 'nobody was listening'. When Stacey told me nobody was listening, she didn't just say it. She almost cried it out, in her gentle, smooth voice, emphasising the disbelief and anger that

'NOBODY... was LISTENING...!' She was trying to be heard, but to no avail. The effect of this was that she felt 'massively out of control' during the birth, and she and her baby were separated after the birth. The real devastation came later. Stacey felt guilty. 'The guilt I felt when I saw (my baby) was AWFUL. I felt like my body had failed her, I wasn't there for her when she needed me. The guilt is still there, every day'.

Stacey's guilt, like a lot of mothers' guilt associated with birth trauma, was about feeling that she should have done something differently during the birth. 'I am angry with myself for not saying no during the birth. If only I could have done something different. I should have stood up to more people'. I hear this so much in my work. There is a wonderful hindsight that replays the event in our minds, and with the freedom of imagination, we imagine it differently to how it actually happened. We imagine it with us having the power, with us reclaiming our power. In our fantasy of how it should have gone, we forcefully tell the staff that this is not okay, we are not accepting this, we need to be listened to and respected. And then we don't understand why it didn't happen that way. After all, we are perfectly capable of speaking up in a meeting, or with our own families, and so on. So why did we not do it when we were having our baby, the most important time of all?

I'll tell you why. In Stacey's case, as in others, it's because power got taken from her. It's the same as someone who has been sexually assaulted not understanding why they 'allowed themselves' to be raped. Stacey was taken by surprise. She did not expect to be subtly ignored, or to be not listened to. She did not expect to feel fear. Fear that those in power, those who she was, in that moment, dependent on for her life, would not prioritise her wellbeing. And when she felt that fear for her life, in the hands of people who had control, her mind and body switched on the evolutionary strategy that basically involves a freeze response. A 'do no more harm' response. A 'don't wind them up any more or I'll really be in trouble' response. This is a subconscious survival strategy – one in which you go for the 'I'll try to keep them sweet rather than fight them' strategy because in that moment, while you are on your back, and they are in uniform, they are more powerful than you.

Stacey knew this at a logical level. She would say 'Yeah, I know it wasn't my fault', but emotionally she still felt guilty about not doing enough. It took time to come to a place where she could know at a much deeper level that her mind and body had responded in the 'wisest' way, that her 'freeze' response had been activated. She could begin to forgive herself. It wasn't her fault. There was a very good reason she had not been more assertive. And it was something that was out of her conscious control, and she should never have been put in that position in the first place.

When the trauma of what had happened began to lift, and Stacey was able to feel more at peace with the sadness of what had happened, she noticed that she was also able to share her story more easily, and hear other people's birth stories, without the pain rearing its head. This is common. When we have been robbed of a good birth experience, it is common to find it really difficult to hear other people's happy stories. You're not alone in this. And it doesn't make you a bad person. So it was for Stacey. She knew she had come a long way in her recovery when she went on holiday a few months later. She told me that she had been sitting by a pool chatting to another holidaymaker. This other holidaymaker was pleasant and friendly, and she was chatting away about a difficult decision that she had to make – whether she should have a third baby. This holidaymaker quipped that 'I should have more really, because I'm so good at birthing them. They just pop out.' Stacey heard this. And she felt amused, entertained, slightly disbelieving at the bizarre nature of the flippant statement. But the old bitterness, sadness, rage, guilt and regret was not there. She knew she had moved on from the trauma of the birth.

Feeling that you should have done more is a common response to birth trauma. Understanding why you did or didn't do something, accepting it, and forgiving yourself for that, is an important part of recovery, in my opinion. Sometimes it takes a therapist to help you to get to that. Hopefully, this book is helping a little too.

WHY DO YOU GO OVER AND OVER WHAT YOU COULD HAVE DONE DIFFERENTLY? THE BRAIN SEARCHING FOR CONTROL

I think the ruminating over 'what I should have done differently' is a way for the brain to make sense of what happened, and gain some sense of control. If I am walking to work, and the pavement gives way under my feet, I fall down and end up in hospital, I really need to know what happened. This is because I need to know whether it might happen again. The brain 'scans' for information to help solve the problem. I need to know if it was the way I was walking, or my shoes, or the pavement, or all pavements, and whether the pavement might still give way, or whether I need to watch out for other pavements, and so on. If I don't know the answers to these things, I can never walk on any pavement ever again! So the brain is adept at going over bad things that happened, and finding out what the causes were, so that we can avoid bad things happening again. It is biased towards working out what *you* could have done differently, because if you know that, then you can protect yourself in the future. In the case of a bad birth, we might rack our brains to work out what went wrong. The easiest things to examine and reach a conclusion about are the ones we could actually control, and that is what we did or didn't do. So this is a common reaction to disaster, designed to help us avoid it in the future. If we cannot work out what went wrong, we feel even more insecure and helpless. Unfortunately, all this is based on the presumption that you had control in the first place, and that you could have done something to avoid it. In an attempt to find something that we could have done differently, I've even heard people blame themselves because they left the house: 'If only I hadn't gone out that morning'. It's not very rational, and it's not very kind to blame ourselves, but your brain will do this automatically. So when you feel that you should have done something different at your birth, please note that this is probably your brain trying to find a way to understand what happened so it can mitigate against it in the future. Your brain is more interested in avoiding bad things happening again, than it is in being kind and rational. So please remember that this is an illusion. It was not your fault that you became a victim of the system. I'll repeat that. It was not your fault.

THE EXAMPLE OF MY CHICKENS: TRIGGERS AND SITUATIONAL ANXIETY

I was in my garden one afternoon. I had let my three chickens loose and they were having a good old scratch and peck in my flower beds. One of them, however, got herself tangled up in the bird net that was protecting my strawberries. Those nets are really tangly! It took me quite a while to disentangle the squawky distressed chicken and set her free again. Poor bird.

A week later, I was gardening again, and I let the chickens loose again. The strawberry patch is on the right-hand side of my garden. There are borders down both sides. The three chickens went up the garden as usual. Two of them went off to the right (they like that side because there's a compost heap there). One of them went to the left. Guess which one?

Yes, you're right. The one that got tangled the week before avoided the right-hand side like the plague. Now a chicken, you understand, does not have powers of reason or deduction, as far as we know. My chicken did not think 'Now, where was that net? I want to make sure I avoid it this time. I'm going to head off to the left and then my chances of getting stuck again are reduced'. Nope. She just got a *feeling of anxiety* at the thought of going to the right. Anxiety serves to help us foresee and avoid danger. And I'm afraid that the part of the brain in the chicken that activates when she feels anxiety and avoids something is a part that humans also possess. It's called the amygdala.

If your amygdala has 'remembered' trauma, it will fire off in the form of anxiety when it is in a similar situation again. Even if there is no logical reason to think that you should be anxious, your brain will fire off anyway, because it works on a 'better safe than sorry' principle. It's trying to protect you from danger. It doesn't care if you feel uncomfortable when you are anxious. Your brain has not 'put the memory away' into the past, and it will keep activating when it experiences anything that vaguely resembles the previous danger. This is known as 'conditioning' or 'being triggered' or 'pattern-matching', according to which model you subscribe to. It's the main reason why you can seem to be fine after a difficult birth, but then anxiety hits you during your next pregnancy. It is very common for people to seek help for a traumatic birth years after the birth – because they come when they get pregnant again. Pregnancy is a kind of trigger – reigniting that scared part of the brain. Lucy's story illustrates this.

LUCY'S PREGNANCY REIGNITED A PREVIOUS BIRTH TRAUMA

Lucy came to me because she was pregnant again after a previous traumatic birth. The first birth had been awful for her. She had had flashbacks every night afterwards, and been very anxious, but after about six months she began to feel better. She enjoyed being a mother, and had managed to get on with her life and put the trauma behind her. As she put it 'Overall, I've done well'. I absolutely agreed with her on this, especially when I heard the details of the birth, and got an idea of how horrific the birth had actually been.

However, when she found out she was pregnant again two years later, the trauma resurfaced. She told me 'I'm not coping well with the planning for this time'. Lucy is a very grounded, rational, emotionally intelligent, confident person. However, when she went to her antenatal appointments, she lost the ability to use these skills of hers, because all she could do was cry. Every time. To add to her difficulties, she was offered a 'debrief session', to go over her notes and try to make some sense of the trauma. However, this made things worse and, in her words, she 'spiralled out'. Her feelings were not attended to, and she was simply shown her medical notes with a view to giving her 'medical insight'. This opened up the old wounds and deepened the trauma. She was not improving. The pregnancy was progressing. In her words, 'I'm stuck, I've got these irrational beliefs, I'm reliving the birth, my mind keeps looping back to it, again and again'.

In a strange kind of way, what happened to my chicken is similar to what was happening in Lucy's brain. The anxiety part of the brain, housed in the amygdala, was triggered when the brain found itself in a similar situation again. This process often means that you can be completely fine after a traumatic event, until something triggers the anxiety. A common example is having to go back to the same hospital where it happened. Here's an example from a post on social media, from a woman who wanted to attend a debrief session, but knew that going into the hospital would trigger her trauma.

In order to have an appointment, they want me to come back to the maternity department. And I just cannot do it. I know that ultimately I need to take a deep breath and find a way to get over such issues. However, in order to make use of such an appointment, I also need to be able to speak coherently and ask the questions I have – and I know that if I force myself to return to the department, I will end up a shaking, crying wreck and completely incoherent, and it would be a waste of their time as well as mine.

While you might not have got PTSD from your difficult birth, you might still have some symptoms of trauma which don't show themselves until you become pregnant again. This effect, just like with my chickens, can happen in all walks of life. One of the most common ways that it presents itself is with a history of childhood trauma. Maybe you buried it well, got on with life, but found it resurfaced during pregnancy and birth. If this happens to you, it can be difficult to understand why you were fine before, but you aren't now. You are not going crazy. It's just your amygdala being reminded of previous dangers, and it is firing off, creating anxiety for you, in a misguided bid to protect you. Psychological therapy can really help with this. For more ideas of how to overcome this effect, see Chapters 4 and 8 on recovery.

THE CASE OF THE AWFUL BACK PAIN: TRAUMA CAN MANIFEST PHYSICALLY

Why is the mind/body connection important for birth trauma? For many reasons, but not least because trauma can manifest physically as well as psychologically. In other words, psychological injury, or trauma, can become evident, or 'play out', in physical ways. It is not often that this relationship is obvious to us, and if we are not looking for it, we might miss it. I think research needs to start asking about it more. There are two anecdotal experiences that I had as a therapist that illustrated it very well for me.

TRAUMA MANIFESTS PHYSICALLY: THE WOMAN WITH DEBILITATING VERTIGO

I was asked to see a woman who was struggling as a result of an accident she had been in. She was crossing a road, when, out of the blue, she was hit by a car. Luckily, she wasn't too badly injured, but she was struggling psychologically. She was a very resilient woman, with a lot of coping strategies and good social and spiritual support. However, this woman was struggling with severe and debilitating vertigo, which meant she could barely stand for long enough to take a shower, and had problems sleeping. She slept upright, her husband had to escort her everywhere, and she could never be left alone in case she toppled over as a result of the vertigo. She had loved to go out shopping on her own, but she was unable to go down her garden path, never mind go on a bus on her own. This was leading to quite a lot of distress, as you can imagine. When I assessed her, I realised that my job was to help her to come to terms with the problem, which the medical community had been unable to treat despite months and months of doctors and hospital appointments. I also assessed for PTSD. She was able to describe the accident without any undue distress, and she wasn't having any nightmares or flashbacks, so I ruled out PTSD. However, I did notice something interesting when she recounted the accident to me. While describing the accident, she said 'I was tossed into the air like a rag'. She told me that she practically landed on her feet, and she walked off with barely a bruise. I asked her about the being 'tossed'. She told me that she remembered the world going 'round and round' (although it was actually her body going round and round). What struck me was that the words she used for the accident were the same words she was using for the vertigo. She had said it felt like her whole body was constantly going 'round and round' and she had a feeling that she wasn't on the ground. So I decided to do a trauma-based treatment with her (the rewind method), even though she had no signs of psychological trauma. One rewind later, and the vertigo began to lift. Within a few weeks, she was bathing on her own, going into town on her own, and very much cheered up!

I believe trauma can manifest physically in the body, without any obvious psychological symptoms. The body can remember, and plays out the symptoms in a physical way. There are many physical treatments and energy treatments out there, which I don't know much about. But if you feel that you would benefit from a physical treatment such as yoga for trauma, or some kind of energy healing, or breath work, or a hands-on therapy, then I would absolutely say go for it. Find someone you trust, or who comes recommended, and see for yourself the benefits of therapies that access trauma through the body. As a clinical psychologist, I do it the other way around. I access physical trauma via psychological therapy. Madeleine's experience of birth trauma is a nice example of this.

THE CASE OF THE EXCRUCIATING BACK PAIN

Madeleine came to me because we were chatting one day about the workshops that I run, training birth workers in the rewind method for lifting birth trauma. She was interested in my work, which I took to be politeness on her part. But it turns out she was genuinely intrigued. She told me that she had had an awful birth, nearly 20 years ago. While she told me the story, I got the feeling that it was still quite raw for her, and that she hadn't ever really got over it. (Later, during our sessions, this was confirmed when she told me that she thought about it every day, that she felt that her body had failed her, that she felt guilty, and that the birth had been a 'complete disaster'.) In an effort to help, I offered to rewind the memory for her. She jumped at the chance. Because we worked in the same building, I happened to know that Madeleine sometimes had excruciating episodes of back pain, which could render her incapacitated for days on end. I said that sometimes I work with managing pain, so we might be able to do something around that too. But it turned out I didn't need to. While preparing to do the rewind with Madeleine, she told me that when she had had her baby, she had experienced a 'white-hot pain... a pain that made me think that I can't possibly experience this level of pain and stay alive through it'. I asked her if it was similar to the back pain she experienced now, 20 years after the birth. She said yes. We did the rewind.

Madeleine's feelings about the birth changed dramatically when the trauma lifted. Where there had been guilt and self-blame, there was now a sense of freedom and lightness, knowing it was not her fault, proud that she had battled through such a brutal process, and lived to nurture and love her son. I had expected that. But I hadn't known whether it might make a difference to her episodes of back pain. I did think there was a possibility that the back pain was a physical manifestation of the birth trauma – that her body remembered the pain, and re-experienced it now and again, a bit like a flashback. Over two years later, Madeleine tells me that she has not had one episode of intense and debilitating pain like she used to do. She tells me that she still gets problems with her back, and that the pain does happen, but it is much milder, and it doesn't prevent her from going about her daily activities. She says 'I know the word "miraculous" is overused by people, but it's what it has been. It was, and it is, miraculous'.

RECOVERING FROM PSYCHOLOGICAL TRAUMA: SELF-HELP

YOUR BRAIN AND BODY ARE DESIGNED TO HEAL

Bad things happen to people. And other mammals. Whether these bad things are physical, or emotional, our bodies and brains are designed and adapted to heal the injury. Let's take an example of a physical injury. If I cut my finger, there is a danger that it won't heal. It might leave a scar, or it might get infected. It might even kill me. But the chances are that it will sort itself out and heal just fine. The body knows how to go about trying to heal itself.

Psychological injury is the same. The brain is designed to heal when bad things happen to us. Some research has tried to put some figures on this, and suggests that for women who have had traumatic births, 62% did not develop any symptoms of PTSD, and of those that did, 18% recovered within six months (Dikmen-Yildiz et al). How does this healing take place, and what can you do to harness it? Well, when we cut our finger, things happen at a biological level that I don't understand – things associated with blood flow, red blood cells, white blood cells, increased blood pressure and so on. But there are also behavioural changes that happen instinctively. We are likely to stop immediately, look at the injury, tell someone, put the fingure in our mouth, or pinch it to stem the bleeding, bandage it and protect it from further injury.

With trauma, there seem to be physical changes taking place in the brain neurologically, but there are also behavioural changes that we do naturally, which are good for us. Firstly, we will seek safety. Once safe, we will likely think back to what happened, analyse it, talk to people about it, dream about it, mull it over, wonder what we could have done differently and so on until we come to terms with what happened. Talking about it seems to help us to recover, as long as we do so voluntarily.

In other words, it is okay to want to talk about it, and it is okay to try to make sense of what happened. Turning to others for social support is a healthy thing to do. It is when we avoid talking about it, and avoid thinking about it, that we may inadvertently interrupt the natural healing process. When we begin to come to terms with what happened, we begin to feel that it is in the past, we are okay now, we are safe now, and it wasn't our fault, or if it was, we can forgive ourselves for the mistakes we may have made. This is a process known as 'reframing' in psychology. It is the ability to shift a negative or limiting view into a more helpful one. For example, I may have felt like my body let me down after a traumatic birth, but I may grow to see that my body was actually strong for surviving the onslaught of a medical birth. In fact, trauma can be so effective in providing a reframing experience for us, that it has a name. Post-traumatic growth.

POST-TRAUMATIC GROWTH: YOU GROW THROUGH WHAT YOU GO THROUGH

When we have experienced something truly awful, there is a capacity not only to heal from it, but also to become stronger.

This ability to come out of adversity with more strength and resilience than we previously had is known as post-traumatic growth. Research suggests that women who experience post-traumatic growth find themselves more appreciative of life, feel that they are stronger as a result of what happened, find that they are more able to draw on the support of others, and gain more from their close relationships. As the old adage goes: you learn who your friends really are.

This post-traumatic growth is part and parcel of reframing the experience – of being able to see that we didn't fail, it wasn't our fault, and that we survived and can go on to thrive. I think it is why it is so healing to turn to others for support: they can help break down any unhelpful beliefs that you may be carrying (such as 'I am weak' or 'I am ashamed') and help you to reframe them into 'I survived' and 'I am a kickass mother' (or whatever might fit for you!). I don't want you to feel any pressure with this one. This reframing doesn't have to be monumental or life-changing. It can just be 'it happened and it was rubbish'. The point is that some people come out of trauma feeling stronger or wiser or more mature. My aim is also that this book will help you to reframe your experience in a more helpful way. Research suggests that being able to reach out to others for support is key in helping turn psychological injury into post-traumatic growth. So don't hesitate to get out there and tell people, talk about it, or just ask them for a hug.

THE CONDITIONS FOR GOOD HEALING

I mentioned earlier that recovery from trauma is similar to recovery from physical injury. Let's look at an analogy with recovery from the common cold. You are likely to get better on your own. Your body will activate your immune system, and get on with the job of killing off the virus that is causing the problem. However, there are things that you can do which will help your body to recover (and things you can do to impede recovery). You would naturally slow down a little, not work too hard, maybe avoid an all-night party, or avoid running a marathon, maybe go to bed a little earlier. These behaviours would increase your chances of healing, and reduce your chances of further injury, such as a chest infection, pneumonia or sepsis. In other words, you are more likely to heal spontaneously, and avoid further damage, if you give your body the best conditions for recovery. It is the same for trauma. Our brains are designed to heal after trauma. And it is more likely to happen if you give yourself the best conditions for recovery. In order to do that, we want you to activate your relaxation/rest and restore system. This is the key to healing. Let's find out more.

FIND YOUR ANTIDOTE: THE REST AND RESTORE SYSTEM

So, you've been psychologically injured by a traumatic event. This means that your stress system is firing away, acting as though you are still in danger, and releasing the hormones associated with that. This 'fight or flight' system is designed to keep you alive, temporarily, in the face of danger, and it doesn't feel good. We have spent a lot of time exploring the fight or flight system, because that is what has been triggered by birth trauma. But what we are now much more interested in is the *antidote* to the fight or flight system.

An antidote is defined as 'something that counteracts an unpleasant feeling or situation'. Isn't that exactly what you would like if you have been traumatised? Absolutely. The antidote to the fight or flight system is another system which is the polar opposite. It is a mechanism which cannot express itself simultaneously with stress. If you enter into it, by definition you come out of the stress system. It is the soothing/compassionate system. It has been called many different things by different authors, such as the rest and restore system, the compassionate system, the tend-and-befriend system, the rest and digest system, the relaxation system, and the affiliative system, among others. This system is one in which your mind and body activate a set of hormones which elicit feelings of calm, relaxation, safeness, playfulness, lovingness, peace. It is associated with being at peace, or feeling grounded, or feeling safe or contented. It is mediated by relaxation and bonding hormones such as oxytocin and endorphins. It is a state in which we tend to feel warmer towards others, or can enjoy their touch and their company more. It is a state in which we tend to want to just 'be' – rather than rush off to do other things. It feels good once we are in it, and we tend to want to just carry on relaxing, maybe similar to a Sunday afternoon on the sofa, or a relaxing morning on a beach on holiday.

Here is a table that shows us the difference between being in your stress system and being in your relaxation system.

Features	Stress 'fight or flight' system	Relaxation 'rest and restore' system
Hormones	Adrenaline, cortisol	Oxytocin, endorphins
Emotions	Fear, stress, distress	Calm, content, relaxed
Physiology	Activated, heart rate goes up	Deactivated, heart rate regulated
Immune system	Put on hold	Works as normal
Digestion	Put on hold	Works as normal
Interpersonal behaviour	Distanced, cold, aggressive	Warm, loving, affiliative
Thinking patterns	Frenetic, negative	Slower, more realistic, open
Motivation	To avoid, escape, fight	To socialise, relax, play, stay put
Mediated by	Sympathetic nervous system	Parasympathetic nervous system

When we are in the soothing 'rest and restore' system, we allow our minds and bodies to begin to heal. In order to recover from your difficult birth, it is important that you pay attention to what calms you, because this is also what will heal you. As you calm, you release the hormones for healing. It's as simple as that! This is why people go on about mindfulness so much, because when we practise mindfulness, we also practise putting our minds into the soothing 'rest and restore' system. Here are some ideas for how you can activate your rest and restore system. Please bear in mind that if you have full-blown PTSD, it might be very difficult indeed to activate your relaxation system with any of the following suggestions. This is not your fault, and I would recommend that you seek the help of a professional to guide you through your recovery. Also, you might find that when you enter your rest and restore system, your anxiety goes up temporarily, and you find that you want to stop. That is okay too – go easy on yourself.

FIND YOUR ANTIDOTE: THINGS YOU CAN DO TO ACTIVATE YOUR HEALING

There are plenty of structured activities which help you to step out of the threat system (fuelled by adrenaline and cortisol), and help you to step into the soothing system (fuelled by endorphins and oxytocin). Almost all alternative therapies have this effect, including reflexology, massage, mindfulness, meditation, aromatherapy, and yoga. It is no coincidence that these originate from the East, where mind and body are viewed as interconnected. Heal the mind, and you heal the body. If you have tried just one of these alternative therapies and liked it, maybe that is the thing to start with now.

I know it's not easy to find the time when you have a baby, but this is important. Some of them are free, and can be done in your own home, maybe via video-link, in just a few minutes. Some of them you will be paying for, such as massage or reflexology. Once again, I would argue that this should be a priority for you: do not feel that you aren't important enough! Your emotional welfare is paramount. You have been through a very difficult birth, and you absolutely matter, more now than ever, because you are a mother.

Even if you know that you want to do more to enter your

rest and restore system, you might find it difficult to actually get around to doing something about it. That is normal. It is because when we are in our threat system, the last thing we are driven to do is to stop and relax! It feels counterintuitive. If feels much more important to get the washing done, or deal with a zillion problems, or make a phone call. You have to overcome this instinct to stay 'stressed', and make yourself do something relaxing, even if you really don't want to. Once you have started to do it, you will notice the benefits, and you will probably not want to stop! Because when we are in the relaxation system, we tend to want to stay there.

CONNECT WITH PEOPLE

People are good for us. Whether in strong, mutual, loving relationships, or just a wave and a hello to a neighbour, positive human interaction is healthy. When you are recovering from an emotional injury such as trauma, or a physical injury for that matter, find ways to include 'people time' in your recovery. You might find that you are distancing yourself from people because you feel they don't understand, or you feel irritable, or you feel ashamed. Try to be aware of this so that you can counteract it.

There is burgeoning science around the power of connection, helping us to see that when we feel supported, loved, connected, safe, and in company, we release hormones that activate our relaxation response, which has an immediate physiological effect on our bodies, reducing our blood pressure, boosting our immune system, regulating our heart beat, activating the parts of our brains associated with calm, and deactivating the stress centres. Ways in which you might do this are numerous. Accepting help is something that people often advise new mothers to do, and I think it is a great tip for many reasons. You get practical help. Hurray. But you also get a sense that people care about you, and that they are there for you. Don't wait for them to offer. People aren't always going to offer: maybe they don't want to intrude, maybe they don't want to offend, maybe they presume you will ask. You need to ask outright. Generally, people love to help, especially when new babies are involved.

Bring people around you who help you feel loved. Show your partner this part of the book, so that he or she understands that they can do a huge amount to help by asking you how you are, making you cups of tea, encouraging you to rest, physically holding you or giving you a hug. You have, in effect, been injured psychologically, so some tender loving care is a part of your prescription. If this becomes a bit of a joke between you, that's fine too. Laughter is healthy. If you haven't got a partner, or the relationship isn't too good, then bring in others. Friends, mothers, health visitors – anyone who you feel will understand and be kind.

FIND YOURSELF SOME PRIVACY

As well as being with people who help you feel loved, it's also important to get some privacy for yourself. Often, mothers struggle to meet this need, and when it isn't met, it can lead to frustration and anxiety, which isn't good if your brain is already at its stress limit due to trauma. My advice is to find a way to get some peace in the day or week. Taking a bath is a common favourite. Or maybe a walk. Locking yourself in the toilet while someone else covers for you. Or simply going to bed early, with a hot chocolate and magazine, and instructions not to be disturbed for a few moments. When you calm your brain, you help to heal your pain.

FOOD AND WATER

Okay, this might seem obvious, but the fact is that when you are a mother, you are more likely to think that the need for good nourishing food is a priority for your baby, but not for you. Grabbing a sandwich? Living off chocolate and coffee? Going thirsty because there are more urgent things to do?

Research shows us that what you eat affects your mood. Good food helps the brain to function better. Okay, so there isn't any evidence (as far as I know) that food can help heal trauma, but if it helps with anxiety, inflammation and tissue recovery, then I am surmising that it helps with psychological trauma too. At the very least, it is true that when we are hungry or thirsty, we release cortisol, which is a stress hormone. So my advice is to think about what you are eating and drinking, and help your mind and body to heal by feeding yourself nourishing foods. Once again, recruit the help of other adults for this – ideally, someone else should be looking out for you here, making sure you have what you want while you are sat feeding, or that something is being prepared while you are grabbing some sleep. Read this part out loud to your partner... it might help!

PRIORITISE SLEEP

Did you know that your body heals while it sleeps? Both physically and psychologically. During those hours snuggled up under your duvet, you might think you are doing nothing, but in fact, while you rest and relax, your body is given the opportunity to get busy. Your body sets about repairing and restoring, encouraging healthy tissue growth, attacking viruses and bacteria, finding and deleting unhealthy tissue, reducing inflammation, and so on. If you are ever guilty of underestimating the importance of sleep in keeping you fit and healthy, just remember that without sleep, we die! That makes it as important as oxygen, food and water for survival.

To keep fit and healthy, both physically and mentally, we need to sleep. In terms of mental health and brain activity, during sleep the brain goes about getting rid of toxins and waste via a system known as the glymphatic system. Not only does the brain clear out toxins, but it also builds and strengthens healthy brain support cells and neural connections while you sleep. Research suggests that this leads to better learning, more balanced emotions, and less anxiety. So it is important to prioritise your sleep. I know that this is difficult with a new baby. It will rely on two things – firstly, good support from other people. Sit them down and delegate ways in which they can help you, so that you can rest more. This might include mothers, fathers, partners, neighbours, friends, nannies, doulas, cleaners. If you find this too awkward, maybe your partner could enable it to happen. The second way to help yourself to sleep is to read up on the new literature and research about co-sleeping and bed-sharing with your baby – especially if you are breastfeeding. This is a game-changer for many parents, because if you know how to rest and sleep safely with your baby, you will naturally feel more settled and relaxed because your baby is close to you, you can hear her, feel her, and you can sleep better because your biological need to be close to her is being met.

Other ways to help you to get more rest and sleep are to practice sleep hygiene. This involves keeping your bedroom dark, comfortable and peaceful at night, so that you and your baby associate it with rest. Even if you aren't sleeping, we want you to be resting and relaxing. Your room should feel good to be in, you should eliminate blue light, and be mindful of how you use your phone at night. I often suggest to mums that they have a special treat next to them at night for when they are feeding their baby – that way, their baby gets to enjoy a feed, and so do you!

It's not just a new baby that can interrupt your bid to get more sleep. Trauma will also interrupt your sleep. If you have been traumatised, your brain will behave as though it is in danger, and mammals do not rest easy when there is danger about! You might have nightmares, and be scared to sleep, or you might find that scary memories come to the surface as soon as you rest your head on your pillow. I'm so sorry if this is happening to you. Recovery is important, so take yours seriously, and things will get better as the trauma heals. There is some evidence that while we are dreaming, our brain is processing the things that have happened to us, so it may be that having nightmares is part of the brain's attempt to heal. This makes intuitive sense, especially given that people often report nightmares soon after a traumatic event, but the frequency and severity of them will fade with time, as the person recovers.

In summary: your physical health and mental health are inextricably linked, and if you want your mind to heal, it really helps to take good care of yourself as a basis for further work. Access all and any alternative therapies such as yoga, massage, reflexology, reiki and so on. Take care of your sleep, diet, and rest well. Connect with those who are good for you, and who support you. Delegate a lot of what you might normally want to do, such as the housework and school runs. I know that there are many practical obstacles to doing this, and that it is very dependent upon finances, and social support. There are psychological obstacles too, like feeling that you 'should' be doing it all, or not being able to ask for help easily, or not realising that you matter too. But you do matter, for the simple reason that you are a mum. You need to put your own oxygen mask on, so that you can help your baby with her oxygen mask. Prioritise your recovery, because when you are well, you can be your very best as a mother. If anyone asks, just tell them that your clinical psychologist has prescribed it for you.

Once you are starting to do what you can to take better care of yourself, it's time to move onto the next two steps in your recovery. They are learning grounding techniques, and using your breath to manage your stress. Let's look at grounding techniques first.

THE IMPORTANCE OF GROUNDING TECHNIQUES

In order to recover from trauma, and to be able to look back on what happened to you without fear and horror, we need you to be able to look at it and still feel safe. We don't want that amygdala to light up too much!

If you have been traumatised, you might find that when you think about the awful memory, your brain seems to drift off into it and get stuck there, like being lost in a thrilling story, or captivating film. Temporarily, your attention is subsumed by the story or the film or the memory. Mentally, you're not actually in the present moment. Before you know it, your heart is racing, you're upset, you're stressed, and feeling awful. Not all that different, in fact, to how you felt during the actual traumatic event. The most severe form of this process is an actual flashback, when your brain temporarily loses touch with the present, and feels like it is reliving the past in its full glory. This feels awful, and it's activating your stress centres. It might happen when you read this book, and as such, it might stop you reading it, and getting the benefit from it. So if you begin to feel very anxious, or panicky, or begin to get too lost in the painful parts of the memory, I advise you to stop and regroup emotionally. This is something that therapists call grounding, and it is a useful skill to learn. It means coming back to the here and now, pulling yourself out of 'daydreaming' mode.

Grounding is not avoidance. It's important to note that there is a difference between grounding yourself and avoidance. I'll give you an analogy. If I were learning to swim, I would not just jump in at the deep end and see what happens. I would make sure that I could touch the bottom when I needed to, and I would make sure that I could get out when I wanted to. But I would need to touch the water. I would not be able to avoid water altogether. It's the same for you. As you recover from your traumatic experience, you do need to touch the memory. You can't avoid it altogether if you want to be able to reach the point where you can look back on it and not feel the horror. But I want you to be able to touch the memory in a way that doesn't feel too scary, and I want you to be able to take a break from the emotions as and when you need to. The grounding techniques and the breathing techniques help you to do just that. Once you can do those, you can go on to try the other do-it-yourself healing techniques that follow.

FOUR WAYS TO GROUND YOURSELF

Here are four of my favourite grounding techniques, though there are many more. Have a go at all of them, and see which suits you best. You will need to practise them, and I suggest you begin to practise them when you are already fairly calm. This is because if you try to use a technique for the first time when your stress levels are really high, there is a chance of the stress winning out, because your brain has evolved to override relaxation when it thinks there is danger. So practise every day while you are fairly relaxed, and then start to apply your favourite ones when you are stressed or can feel the traumatic memory taking over.

1 'BLINK YOUR EYES, SQUEEZE YOUR HANDS AND WIGGLE YOUR TOES'

Open your eyes, if you haven't already. Then blink twice. Notice your eyelashes move. Then drop your attention down to your hands. Look at them. Where are they? Resting, maybe on the bed, or on your lap? Squeeze them into fists lightly, and let go. Then look to your feet. Notice where they are resting on the bed, or on the floor. Notice the bed or the floor underneath your feet. Wiggle your toes. You can keep moving between blinking your eyes, squeezing your hands, and wiggling your toes, until you feel grounded again.

2 'I CAN SEE, HEAR AND FEEL'

Open your eyes, if you haven't already. Notice and identify three things that you can see in your room. Name them. Then move your attention to sounds around you. Notice three things you can hear. Take your time, the sounds will come. Name them. Then move your attention to three things that you can feel – maybe your feet resting, or the warmth of the room, or your breathing. That's great. You're going to go back and do that again, but drop it to two things that you can see, two things you can hear and two things you can feel. They can be new things, or they can be the same as before. Then, do that again, but with only one thing that you can see, one thing you can hear and one thing you can feel. At the end of this, you should notice that you are much calmer in yourself.

3 'I LIKE TO MOVE IT, MOVE IT'

Some people, when they get stressed, find a strong urge to move. This makes sense in terms of the fight/flight reaction. With this exercise, we want the movements to be mindful and calm, rather than jerky and stressed. When done calmly, movement is a very powerful relaxation tool. You might try standing up, and stretching your arms up over your head, and get up on your tiptoes. Hold the stretch for a moment, and then, with a nice long breath out, bring your arms slowly back down to your sides, and bring your feet down flat again. Do that again, and do it nice and slowly so that you have time to notice how it feels to make those movements. Staying in touch with how it feels is the aim, and this can be a little challenging because you might find your mind wandering aimlessly. That's fine: if that does happen, just notice, before bringing your mind back to what it feels like to be moving your body. Moving your body, reconnecting mindfully with your body, and releasing stress and trauma through body movements is something that yoga specialises in. If you think that yoga might be for you, don't hesitate to find a local practitioner near you.

4 THE OLD-FASHIONED FAVOURITE: DISTRACTION

In my practice, I find that many people intuitively use distraction as a way to calm themselves down when they are getting distressed. This is simply the art of making yourself think about something completely different, or do something that will interrupt your train of thought. For example, texting a friend, putting on a piece of music, watching an old favourite TV programme, doing something physical such as cleaning, taking the dog for a walk, going to the local shop, and so on.

BREATHING AND MINDFULNESS TECHNIQUES: YOUR BREATH IS THE KEY TO YOUR STRESS

Did you know that how you breathe has a direct link to your stress system? When you get stressed, your breathing changes, your heart rate changes, your heart rate variability changes, your hormones change, your blood pressure changes and so on. But the only one of these that you can directly and consciously change is your breathing. It's a powerful tool to helping you activate your rest and restore system. It is worth spending some time learning how to change your breathing to change your stress. If you are a human being, it will work! There are four simple but powerful breathing and mindfulness techniques for you to try. We'll take them one at a time, but the goal is to use them all in unison.

1 MINDFUL BREATH

You breathe every minute of every day, and you always have done. That is obvious, because otherwise you would be dead. But how often do you ever actually *notice* your breathing? If you have had a panic attack in the past, you probably noticed it then, but other than that, it's likely that you never pay any attention to your breath. Being mindful of your breath is a really nice way to enter your relaxation system. Here's how to do it:

HOW TO DO MINDFUL BREATHING

Get yourself comfortable. Make a mental note of how relaxed you feel right now – maybe rate it from a zero (super relaxed) to 10 (anxious). Take in a slow deep breath through your nose, and then let out a lovely, long,

---

slow breath, out through your mouth. Do that again. Close your eyes (optional). Now, revert to your normal breathing rhythm – don't make any attempts to change it, just breathe normally. What you are going to do is *pay attention to what it feels like*. Simple as that. Notice your breaths in, notice your breaths out. Now, begin to notice movements in your body that accompany your breath – maybe in your shoulders, or your ribcage. Maybe your shoulder blades, or your abdomen. Notice that the air feels cooler as you breathe in, and warmer as you breathe out. Did you ever notice that before? Notice how the breath feels as it enters your nostrils or your mouth. Notice it as it moves down into your lungs. Notice the way that your breath seems to pause briefly when you reach the top of your breath, before breathing out again. After at least a couple of minutes of doing this, make another mental note, rating your relaxation levels from zero to 10. If it is less, well done. You have just managed to make some significant and health-giving physiological changes to your body. Your mind and body will thank you if you do this more regularly. If your anxiety is higher, I would suggest you move on to try another breathing technique.

2 REGULATED OUT-BREATH, OR 7–11 BREATH

While you were doing your mindful breathing, you may have noticed that it is the outbreath that relaxes you. A nice long outbreath sends a message to the body that 'all is well'. It regulates our heart rate, which also creates calm in the body. This kind of makes sense, because when danger is over, we 'breathe out a sigh of relief'. Or when we settle down in comfort on the sofa after a hard day, we might intuitively snuggle down with a nice, long, satisfied breath out with a sigh. By contrast, the in-breath is the opposite. We tend to 'gasp' when shocked, or hold our breath when full of anticipation. This is because the body is preparing for action by taking in oxygen to fuel our muscles. Here's the thing – up to now, your mindset has changed your breathing without you realising it. You can now turn this around, and control your breathing to change your mindset. Take control of your breathing to control your levels of relaxation, because when you breathe out more than in, and when you regulate your breath, it sends a message to the brain that all is well. It's kind of a way to convince your mind that it doesn't need to worry right now. Here's how to do it.

HOW TO DO THE REGULATED OUTBREATH, OR 7–11 BREATH

Get yourself comfortable. Make a mental note of how relaxed you feel right now – maybe rate it from a zero (super relaxed) to 10 (anxious). Close your eyes (optional). Take in a slow deep breath through your nose, and then let out a lovely, long, slow breath, out through your mouth. Do that again. You might already notice that it is the outbreath that relaxes you. As you make the outbreath longer, and slower, you become calmer. Great. Do that again. And again. Take your time, stay comfortable while you are doing this. Lovely long breaths out. Keep that pattern of breathing going. Now, you might want to add a count to your breathing. Breathe in for a count of 7, breathe out for a count of 11. Notice the soothing effect of your rhythmic breathing; notice that the counting also creates a sense of relaxation for you. Do this for at least a couple of minutes, and when you're done, make another mental note, rating your relaxation levels from zero to 10. If it is less, well done. You have just managed to make some significant and health-giving physiological changes to your body. Your mind and body will thank you if you do this more regularly. If your anxiety is higher, I would suggest you move on to try another breathing technique.

3 BELLY BREATH

Have you ever watched your baby or toddler sleeping? You may have noticed that their cute bellies move an incredible amount while they sleep, but their ribcage barely moves at all. It's fascinating to watch. This is relaxed breathing at its finest. The reason the belly is moving is that the diaphragm (which is a muscle between your lungs and your abdomen) is moving smoothly and easily with each breath. When we are stressed, our muscles tend to tense up, including the diaphragm. When relaxed, muscles tend to be relaxed too. As you take in air, the diaphragm moves down towards the belly, allowing the air to flow into the lungs and your belly to expand with the push of the diaphragm. When you are relaxed, the diaphragm contracts and expands smoothly with each breath. As we grow older, and face the stresses of modern life more and more, we tend to lose the natural capacity for relaxed belly breathing. This is a shame, because belly breathing sends a message to the brain that all is well. Here's how to do it.

HOW TO DO BELLY BREATHING

Get yourself comfortable. This works better when you're lying down, but you can also do it sitting up, as long as you aren't too scrunched up. Place your left hand on the upper half of your rib-cage. Place your right hand just below your belly button. Make a mental note of how relaxed you feel right now – maybe rate it from a zero (super relaxed) to 10 (anxious). Close your eyes (optional). Take in a slow deep breath through your nose, and then let out a lovely, long, slow breath, out through your mouth. Notice the movements of your hands. You are going to aim, slowly but surely, to ensure that the hand on your belly is moving up when you breathe in, and down when you breathe out. You are aiming for the hand on your ribcage to remain still. You can have a bit of a play with this, experiment a little, maybe exaggerate the movement of your belly as you learn to do this. It will get easier. Be careful not to spend too much time breathing in whilst you do this, or you might end up feeling light-headed. Pay as much attention to your outbreath, as you do to your in-breath, ideally you want your outbreath to be longer than your in-breath. Pay as much attention to getting your belly to sink with the outbreath, as you spend trying to get it to rise with the in-breath. Do this for at least a couple of minutes, and when you're done, make another mental note, rating your relaxation levels from zero to 10. If it is less, well done. You have just managed to make some significant and health-giving physiological changes to your body. Keep practising, and your mind and body will thank you for it.

Your breath is the key to your stress because every time you take control of your breathing, you send a message to your nervous system that all is well, and this calms your nervous system down a little. Start practising the techniques while you feel okay. Don't make the mistake of only trying them out when you are very stressed or when your anxiety has been triggered. It won't work. You need to get good at them beforehand, while you are calm, and you need to practise regularly. It only takes two minutes a day. Maybe do it while you wait for the kettle to boil, or while you are waiting at traffic lights (don't close your eyes, obviously) or before you brush your teeth every day.

Routine is key to being successful with your practice. Once you have practised and got really proficient, you will then be able to use the techniques when you actually need to, and calm yourself down with great effect.

4 PRACTISE MINDFULNESS

Mindfulness is an antidote to our thinking/logical/anxious brain. Mindfulness has been shown to be very effective in helping us manage our anxiety and stress. It is the practice of keeping the stream of our thoughts in the here and now – thereby moving away from the constant stream of future and past thinking which is more likely to involve stress or having a busy mind. When we stay in the present moment, our brain calms down. Hormones are released that are calming. Our heart rate slows, our breathing regulates.

As humans, we can all learn to have more control over what our 'new' brain elicits, thereby controlling the otherwise constant stream of worries, concerns, what ifs, plans, ruminations and so on. Once we step back from engaging with our anxious stream of thoughts (they will probably continue to happen, but we don't buy into it so much), and when we focus on how it feels to be in the here and now, we calm ourselves down. There are many useful phone apps out there, so explore and find one which works for you.

The mindful breathing technique outlined above is a good place to start. But you can be mindful when focusing on any activity. It doesn't have to be about you breathing. For example, you can be mindful while you eat. In doing so, you would focus on the act of eating, and what you can feel/taste/smell/see while you are doing it. It is amazing how much information there is going on while you just put a forkful of food into your mouth. Notice the sensations on your tongue, the texture, the movement of your jaw, the sound in your ears and so on. Usually, our conscious attention filters all this out while we 'think' about stuff in our past or future. When you do the opposite, and attend to the present moment, time seems to stand still, and you begin to slow yourself down, increasing the chances of entering into the relaxation system. You can feel the benefit of this by just doing it for 60 seconds every day. The interesting thing is that if you are stressed or busy, you won't *want* to do it. But when you *make* yourself do it, you then find that time slows down, and nothing seems to be as urgent as you thought it was after all. I like to do this in the shower, and feel the water on my face. You might choose to do it when feeding your baby. Notice the expression on their face. Notice the tiny movements as they drink. Notice the smell of your baby. Notice how your baby feels in your arms. You can choose any time in the day to practise this, and making it into a habit is always a good idea to ensure regular practice.

Having learnt and practised ways of grounding yourself, and ways of activating your relaxation response, you will then be ready to move onto the third stage of do-it-yourself healing: processing.

HOW TO PROCESS YOUR TRAUMATIC BIRTH

Most psychological treatments for trauma involve helping a person to think and/or talk about what happened until they can do so without feeling the accompanying distress associated with the memory. This is sometimes termed 'processing' the memory. I said earlier that in most instances, healing takes place naturally. Have you noticed that you wanted to talk about the birth after it happened? Maybe you still do now. If so, this is healthy. It can be difficult to find the right person to listen, because you have probably been told that it's time to move on from that now, and be grateful. This silences you. But don't give up. It would seem that as long as you choose to do it (don't force yourself) and as long as you can find a kind listening ear, talking about it is good for you. Even if you find it difficult. Especially if you find it difficult.

Telling your story can be an important part of recovery. Bear in mind that telling your story can retrigger the *fear* of the trauma, and we don't want this to happen. We want the fear centres in your brain (your amygdala) to stay reasonably calm to avoid a flashback. If you feel a great deal of fear or distress, I'd advise you to stop, ground yourself and take a break. There is no rush. Having said that, it is only really intense fear and distress I am talking about here. Other emotions, such as lots of tears or lots of sadness, are probably cathartic rather than scary. Allow the tears to flow by all means if that feels at some level that it is healing for you. There are many ways to process your memory, and I will go through some of them with you.

1 WRITE IT DOWN

Often, the process of writing your birth story down on paper can be very therapeutic. It's not clear why, but I presume it has something to do with helping you to make sense of what happened. Neurologically speaking, it is helping your thinking brain to get on board with your emotional brain. It is also, no doubt, helping you to face parts of the memory which you might be avoiding. Intuitively, the process of writing it down on paper creates a sense that you have now got it out of your head.

I have worked with many women who have said that once they had written their story down, they felt a lot better. When you are writing, it can help to include not only *what* happened (it may be that you aren't actually very clear on exactly what happened anyway), but also how you *felt* and what you *thought* during the birth. This is usually where the horror lies, and is usually the part that could do with the attention. Take your time writing it. You might find that it all comes out in one big go. Or you might find that you need to keep taking breaks because it is emotionally draining. If writing your story down is creating a great deal of anxiety, my advice would be to put your pen down and try again another day. There is no rush to do this. Take your time, go easy on yourself.

When you have written your story, it is up to you what you actually do with it. You can plan to destroy it after you have written it, or keep it somewhere special, or share it with someone.

2 WRITE A LETTER

It can also be useful to get your feelings down on paper by writing an imaginary letter to someone that is meaningful to your birth. By imaginary, I mean that you might not actually send it, but just writing it can help process some of your difficult feelings. For example, it might be to someone that you feel let down by, or angry with. It could be to your baby, explaining how you feel, and voicing what you would like to be able to say to your baby. It could even be to your body, and how you feel about what happened. Writing down how you feel is key here, and you can choose to destroy the letter once you've written it. Some people destroy them with great gusto – either ripping them up, or burning them. Remember to take care of yourself here and go easy. If your anxiety or fear escalates, take a break, and ground yourself.

3 DRAW IT OUT

I am not a drawer! But you may well be. When I say a drawer, I don't mean someone who is good at drawing; I mean someone who finds it helpful to express themselves through artwork and drawing. Scribbling, splattering, making shapes, using colours, with paint, pencil, or modelling clay – it doesn't matter. What matters is that you express your feelings around your birth in a form other than words and sentences. Being able to do something creative using your hands alongside something emotional can be very therapeutic. Once again, when it is done, you can choose to destroy it deliberately with purpose. Most people choose to keep it, as a symbol of their struggle and their journey through the healing process.

4 TELL A FRIEND

Sometimes I meet women years after their difficult births, and I ask them 'Have you ever told anyone in detail what actually happened to you?' They think about it, and then they say 'No, I don't think I ever have'. You might have shared bits and pieces of information. But have you actually gone through the birth in detail? If not, you might find it really useful to do so. Find a friend who you think would be helpful to you and willing to listen. Put an afternoon or evening aside to tell them your story. When we chat, we naturally engage in turn-taking, but you will have explicitly asked her to listen to your story in its entirety, so that even if you do turn-take with talking, the understanding is that the conversation will be directed back to your birth and what actually happened. This is a great way to feel heard, and to get the story out of your head and somewhere else.

5 BOUNDARY IT

This is a technique that can be useful for managing rumination symptoms. If your memory of the birth is popping up when you don't want it to, or whizzing around and around in your head and you feel you're going round in circles and can't put a stop to it, then you might like to try this little technique for managing it. This technique aims to help you feel that you are controlling when and if you think about the birth, and not the other way around. Basically, you are going to 'hear it out' by giving it an allotted 'attention time' once a day and sticking to it.

It works like this. Decide when you are going to set aside between 10 minutes and 30 minutes in your day. It might be at 5.30pm before tea, or 7.30pm when your partner gets home, or any other time to suit you. During the day, if you find yourself thinking about it when you didn't want to, tell yourself that it can wait until your next 'attention time'. Then, when the time comes, set up the stopwatch on your phone. Set the timer to the allotted time (between 10 minutes and 30 minutes). Devote that time to *only* thinking about the birth. You can write if you like, or just think. If your mind wanders onto something else, bring it back to the birth. Keep on track – only think about the birth until your time is up. This reverse psychology works really well, because the more you try to stay on task, the more your mind will find it hard to ruminate on the subject in hand. When your time is up, you're done! Get on and do something else. Next time the rumination starts, just remind yourself that it can wait until your next 'attention time'. Over a few days, your brain will adapt and you'll find yourself ruminating much less.

6 DO-IT-YOURSELF THERAPY

I have taken you through some of the usual steps that a therapist might take you through when you begin therapy for trauma. These include grounding techniques, breathing for relaxation, self-care techniques, and ways to process the trauma. Here are a few other things that might happen in therapy, but that you can have a go at yourself. Firstly, letting go of some of the self-blame, shame and guilt that you might be feeling.

LETTING GO OF ANY SELF-BLAME, SHAME OR GUILT

This is a key part of recovery. Give it your due care and attention. Examine to what extent you blame yourself. There are a number of reasons why it is very common to blame yourself following a traumatic birth. You may absolutely believe that you were completely to blame for what happened. You may partly blame yourself and partly blame others. You might realise at a logical level that you were not actually to blame, but you still feel guilty and responsible. What we know logically and how we feel can often be contradictory. You might *know* that you weren't responsible for what happened at the birth, but still *feel* to blame for how you are feeling as a result of the birth. Your emotional mind and your logical mind are not in sync. There is a small chance that it is obvious that you should have done something differently. However, in almost all of these cases, it turns out that hindsight is a factor here. Ask yourself – why did I *not* do what I thought I should have done? There will be a good reason. For example, if I drop a very valuable vase and it smashes, it is true that I should have carried it more carefully. However, the reason I did *not* carry it carefully is important. Maybe I thought it was going in the recycling and didn't realise it was valuable. Maybe I had been drugged without realising. Maybe I heard my child cry out, which distracted me. Maybe there was a kink in the carpet so I lost my balance. Asking yourself *why* you didn't do what you wish you had done, will often help you to see that without the benefit of hindsight, you couldn't have done it any differently! In almost all cases that I have worked with, the mother has felt guilty and responsible, but she comes to realise that she just did her best, and that that was all she could do without the benefit of hindsight.

Self-blame often accompanies a tendency to be self-critical, or unkind to ourselves, or expect much more of ourselves than we would of others. In fact, research has shown that being highly self-critical is a common factor in many mental health problems. We know that people who are kinder to themselves fare better. Cognitive behavioural therapy will often try to work with self-blame, self-criticism and shame, and I'm going to introduce you to a few of the techniques here so that you can try some of them for yourself. They include the friend technique, engaging your compassionate mind, the affirmations technique, and the responsibility pie chart. These techniques can be used for any aspect in which you are struggling psychologically.

THE FRIEND TECHNIQUE

We are generally much harsher with ourselves than we are with others. Have a think about what your 'self-talk' is, or what your private beliefs are, about what happened to you and what you believe that says about you. It can really help to write these down. You may already be painfully aware of what these are, or you may not realise the extent of them. If becoming aware of them is emotionally tough for you, go easy on yourself. It can be quite difficult, and take a little time, to begin to become consciously aware of them. I'll give you an example to help you get an idea of what I mean. It is common to have thoughts similar to the following: 'I failed to birth my baby, why can't I just get over it like other people do? I should be able to just move on, I'm a rubbish mother because I couldn't breastfeed properly, other people can do it, why can't I? There's something wrong with me. I don't deserve to be a mother'. These words hurt, and they don't hurt any less just because you are saying them to yourself. On the contrary, it is much harder to bat them off if we are saying them to ourselves!

The friend technique goes like this. Imagine that you have a friend who you know well, and care for. Imagine that she had been through what you have been through. How would you feel towards her? Would you tell her the same things you tell yourself? If not, why not? If she was telling you that she had failed and that it was her fault, would you secretly agree with her? The chances are you would not. You would know that it would be an even bigger injustice to her to suggest that it was her own fault that she suffered. You would not tell her it is her fault, because you would not want to be unkind. Did you want to be unkind to yourself? If you would not be cruel to her, then please don't be cruel to yourself. You are guilty of only one thing – being unfairly harsh on yourself. Now write down all the things you might say to her, and apply them to yourself. Be careful to use the same tone of voice with your internal self-talk as you would use when talking to her. The chances are you are much gentler with her. You'll need to do this often to help your brain to actually assimilate this, but over time, you should find that you blame yourself less and less, and treat yourself more kindly, because your feelings matter as much as your friend's do.

ENGAGE YOUR COMPASSIONATE MIND

This technique crosses over a little with the friend technique, but instead of focusing on kind *words* that we might say to ourselves, we focus on kind *feelings* towards ourselves. When I feel bad or ashamed, what I actually often need is just a hug. Or acceptance. Or to know that I am loved, and that my mistakes are simply a part of being human and they don't make me a bad person. But what I might do to myself is exactly the opposite. Instead of forgiving and accepting myself, I might chastise and hate myself. This will make me feel worse. This technique involves *imagining* being treated in a loving, accepting way. Imagining it creates changes in your brain that release hormones, that help you to feel better – that's a fact that we know from neuroscience. It's a piece of magic that you can learn to do for yourself. You can choose who or what is going to be your loving, compassionate other. It might be your dog. It might be God. It might be your grandmother. It might be someone imaginary. You can basically create any imaginary being at all; the only rule is that they know you, love you, accept you and that you value their judgement. When you have an idea of the kind of compassionate other you want to imagine, you can focus on all of your senses – sight, sound, feel and smell. You might focus on how they look (a warm smile maybe) or the tone of their voice (perhaps gentle but firm), or the feel of them (warm arms wrapped around you) or even their smell. Try different ways of doing this, be creative, have a play with it. When you do it, spend at least one minute doing it, and notice how it shifts how you feel, even if just temporarily. The more you practise, the better you will be at taking the edge off that nasty feeling of self-blame or shame.

THE AFFIRMATIONS TECHNIQUE

Affirmations are a nice way of affirming and strengthening what you already know, or giving it more power to help you, or consolidating what you are trying to achieve. For example, if you know at a logical level that you were not to blame for your birth being traumatic, but you sometimes still feel as though you were to blame, affirmations can help shift the balance over. All you do is write down what it is you want to believe. In this example, you might write 'I know that I did all I could do at the time' 'I did not deserve to suffer like I did' 'I did my best' 'I was strong for surviving what I survived' 'It is okay to feel upset about what happened' 'I know logically that it was not my fault'. You can write one strong affirmation and stick to that, or you can write a load of them down. It's up to you. Don't write down ones that are miles away from what you can actually believe, because that will backfire. Make sure they are kind too. Once you have written them down, you then need to expose yourself to them daily. You can do this by pinning them up on the bathroom cabinet or on your fridge, or you can have them ping up on your phone as reminders every day. You can decide to read them out loud to yourself once a day – maybe before you brush your teeth, so that you get some routine going with it. Repetition is key here. Keep doing it, and over time, it will become integrated into a natural way of thinking, replacing the old negative and hurtful stuff with more realistic and helpful ways of thinking.

THE RESPONSIBILITY PIE CHART

This is a technique that I use specifically for getting a feeling of guilt into perspective. It can also work if you are angry with your partner or your birth professional for doing or not doing something at the birth that contributed to your distress. If you feel overwhelmed with guilt, and feel that it was your fault that the birth went the way it did, then try this. Draw a circle about the size of an orange on a piece of paper. This is going to be your pie chart of responsibility. You will divide up all the factors that played a role into slices of your circle, like a cake (or pie!). Then brainstorm a list of all the people and things that were involved in your birth. This could include a doctor, a taxi driver, a midwife, another midwife, your partner, your mother, the hospital equipment, your antenatal teacher, a book you read, the manager of the hospital, the NHS, racism, yourself, your baby, your manager, your sister and so on. Make sure you spend time thinking of all the possibilities. Now, work out which ones on your list had any responsibility at all, no matter how small, for what happened. Then decide how much of that pie chart you will allocate to that factor. Maybe you think the midwife was 50% responsible for what happened. And maybe Mother Nature gets 30%. And maybe your partner gets 5%. And maybe the media gets 30%. And maybe the system of changing midwives every 12 hours gets 40%. How much do you get? This will help to clarify that it can't have all been your fault: there were many factors at play, most of which you could not control.

Another method for letting go of an over-inflated sense of responsibility is to ask yourself at which point *exactly* would you have done it differently – you are not allowed the benefit of hindsight for this. You can only go on what you knew at the time. At which point exactly would you have done it differently? Without hindsight, I would imagine you can't pinpoint the exact moment, because with what you knew at the time, you were already doing the best that you could.

RE-PATTERN THE MEMORY WITH THIS DO-IT-YOURSELF NLP TECHNIQUE

The rewind method is a tool which I use in my therapy very often, and I wouldn't be without it when working with trauma. It is part of my therapy package, but it can be used as a tool in its own right. This method has been called different things, such as the visual-kinaesthetic dissociation technique or the fast phobia cure, and it is a tool that has been used by hypnotherapists and Neuro-linguistic programming (NLP) practitioners for decades. It takes many different forms, and is being used by some midwives and other birth professionals across the country to help people overcome the emotional impact of difficult births. It is designed to help your mind to process the uncomfortable feeling associated with the memory. I have adapted it slightly, so that you can do a version of it yourself. If you find that you are constantly thinking about the birth, and cannot stop going over and over it, then this exercise might help you. If, on the other hand, you generally avoid thinking about the memory, or if you think you meet the criteria for PTSD, or if you are having flashbacks and nightmares, please do not try this at home. The way it seems to work is that it gets your brain to remember the traumatic memory in a way that it never has before, and this helps the brain to process the memory in the logical, historical part of your memory, rather than the emotional part of your memory. You will visualise the incident when you are relaxed (for the first time), you will visualise it as though you were looking at yourself (rather than through your own eyes, for the first time) and you will imagine it all backwards (for the first time). Those three different aspects seem to have the magical effect of lifting a lot of the distressing amygdala activity, and helping you to remember it without the old distress. If you decide to give this a go, it is really important that you go carefully. Be clear with yourself, that you can stop whenever you want to, just by opening your eyes. Remember that this may help you if you already find yourself thinking about the memory over and over again, and not to try it if you get flashbacks, or avoid thinking about it.

Here's how you do it:

1 Firstly, you want to be comfortable, free from the chance of disturbance, and relaxed. How you get relaxed is up to you. You can engage the breathing techniques that I outline above, or you could listen to a nice relaxation track, or you could spend some time imagining yourself on your favourite relaxing holiday. Throughout this method, you are going to be pretty chilled. (If you start to get stressed, then take a break. It is important to remember that you can stop and open your eyes at any point that you wish to. Do not do this if you feel anxious, and if you begin to feel anxious whilst you are doing it, then remind yourself that you can open your eyes and stop at any point that you want to).

2 Once you are relaxed, imagine yourself sitting in a very private, comfortable, beautiful cinema. As you sit there, bring to mind a time when you felt confident and assured in yourself, and allow that feeling to flow through you now. You feel safe, confident and assured.

3 In a moment (in step 6), you will imagine a small, black and white film, of the traumatic memory playing on the screen, but it will be slightly different. It will be like an old film, it will be in black and white, and it will have funny piano music playing over it, like old films used to do. It is important that the starting point of the film will be before anything started to go wrong – a time when you felt safe and all was well. It will play through what happened to you, and finish after it was all over, when you knew you were safe again. Remember that you will be watching it like a film, not through your eyes – so this will be a different way of experiencing the memory.

4 Imagine that behind you in this safe, private and comfortable cinema, is a projection room. Imagine yourself floating up from your comfy seat and into that projection room, so that you can look down at yourself sitting in that cinema. You can see how comfortable and safe and confident you are down there. The film is going to play with you watching yourself watching the film from the projection room. When the film is finished, it will stop on a freeze-frame, after it was all over and you knew you were safe again.

5 Just before we run the film, get back in touch with a feeling of strength, ability, pride or power. Think of a time when you did something that made you feel really good. Maybe baking a cake, or winning at sports, or succeeding at something. Let that feeling permeate your entire body, making it stronger, enjoying that feeling, letting it flow through you.

6 It is important to remind yourself that at any point that you want to, you can just open your eyes and come back to the room. From your projection room, let the film play forwards, in black and white, with the music playing, and watch yourself sitting in the cinema, relaxed and watching the screen. Let it play to the very end, when it was all over and you were safe again, and then freeze-frame the picture.

7 Well done. Now, imagine yourself floating out of the projection room and into the screen, so that you are now seeing it through your eyes. In a moment, the film will run backwards very fast, within 1 or 2 seconds, like a fast rewind. So when you're ready, rewind the film, with you in it, superfast, all the way back to the very beginning when all was well.

8 Brilliant. Open your eyes. How do you feel? If you feel kind of good, you can test this now – when you think back to the old traumatic memory, how do you feel? The level of distress will probably have dropped. If so, you can just keep doing this – do it for various parts of the memory, at different speeds, over and over if you like. Every time you do it, you will be diminishing your old fear response as the memory gets processed and transferred from the fear parts of your brain (the amygdala) to the long-term memory parts of the brain in the neo-cortex.

TAP IT OUT WITH DO-IT-YOURSELF EFT

EFT stands for Emotional Freedom Technique. It's sometimes known as the tapping technique. The idea is that you tap on certain meridian points on the body, or energy points, while paying attention to the emotion that is bothering you. Arguably, EFT creates a form of dissociation while you focus on the distress, which, interestingly, also happens during other trauma treatments, such as the Rewind method and EMDR (Eye-Movement Desensitisation and Reprocessing). The NHS doesn't endorse it, and I am not trained in it and don't know much about it, but I've heard very good things anecdotally. Tricia Murray is an EFT practitioner, and she told me that she uses it for herself to great effect:

As a woman who has experienced anxiety and low mood for most of her life, EFT was the tool that changed me. I didn't need to go into a dark room with headphones or time to unwind to meditate or practice mindfulness. All those approaches are brilliant but when you have an anxious brain, sometimes you can get more anxious and cross with yourself because you can't settle into meditation. I've loved the physical aspect of tapping on myself and been able to use it for all sorts of things. My whole family have benefitted at times when they've been unsettled, stressed and anxious. I love hearing my kids trying to teach their friends tapping, or being able to settle my baby when he's overtired using very gentle tapping on some of the points.

I have had a dabble in EFT for personal use, and found it quite powerful. Tricia goes on to say:

EFT works like other talking therapies and at the same time stimulating various points on the hands, head, face and body through tapping. These points regulate the nervous system and elicit a sense of calm in the body. Through this process, the person feels calm when they bring to mind the issue. It can be used both as a self-help tool or as a therapeutic intervention depending on the severity of what the person needs help with.

If your trauma or anxiety are particularly bad, or you meet the criteria for PTSD, seek the help of a professional. If you do decide to have a go yourself, it is easy to learn to do, using videos from the internet. It can release some strong emotions, such as anger, grief, and shame, and you might find that you move through all of these emotions as you tap, but I think that is part of the process of recovery. If you do give it a go, pay attention to the 'mantra' that you give yourself while you tap. In its simplest form, your mantra will be 'Even though I had an awful birth, I fully and completely accept myself'. This can change as you move through the emotions, and you might find yourself using 'Even though I feel ashamed about my birth, I fully and completely accept myself' or 'Even though I am angry at the doctor, I fully and completely accept myself'.

I'm hoping that what you have gained from this chapter is some insight into practical ways in which you can facilitate your natural recovery from your ordeal, and some specific ideas that you might like to try. But recovery isn't just about specific techniques. It's also about coming to a place of understanding and acceptance. Hopefully the book as a whole will help you to understand your situation a little better, let go of some of the guilt or confusion, and help you see that your trauma is not your fault or a sign of weakness.

However, sometimes, the injury is one for which self-help, care and understanding is not enough. Sometimes, whether it be for a cut on our finger that has gone septic, a cold that has turned into pneumonia, or a bad birth that has turned into full-blown PTSD, we need an expert to help us recover. If you find it extremely difficult or impossible to do any of the techniques in this chapter, because they elicit terror or avoidance or flashbacks, or if you've tried any of them and it seems to have made things worse, then I would suggest you have a think about getting some expert help to recover. Treatments are very effective these days, and can turn your life around. I describe some of them in Chapter 8.

– 5 –

FAMILIES AND PARTNERS: HOW YOU CAN HELP

Emotional support makes a difference to how we manage emotional problems. When trauma comes into the mix, it can be really difficult to know how to ask for support, or for people to know how to support you. This chapter helps your loved ones to understand trauma, and how to help. Why not pass the book onto them and ask them to read this chapter, as a great way to let them know that you value their support? Let them know that you are asking them to read this because they matter in your life.

Being the partner or parent of someone who is struggling with trauma is not easy. The person that you love doesn't have a broken arm, or a gash to the head, or a limp, to help you *see* that they are actually suffering. If you have not suffered with trauma before, or even anxiety or depression, it is almost impossible to understand how they feel. It can be almost impossible to know how to help. If you want to help, that is a great start. This chapter will give you some guidance on how you might do that. This chapter applies to partners of mothers who have been traumatised, but I am also talking to birth mothers whose partners have been traumatised by the birth. As we see in Chapter 6, fathers and partners can be traumatised too.

The first thing I want you to know is this: *you are the unsung hero in all of this.* Living with someone with PTSD is not easy: you go through pain, you see it, you experience it, you have to deal with it moment by moment, but you don't get to leave it at the end of the day, you don't have the expertise or the knowledge to know what to do, no one is there to check that you are okay, or that you are coping. You are living with uncertainty, unpredictability and a constant feeling that you don't really know whether you're doing it right or not. The thing is, and I want you to feel good about this (rather than pressured by it): you can make a huge difference. Research shows that your help is very important, because feeling supported is a big factor in people recovering from perinatal mental health problems. We know that feeling alone or isolated or unsupported is associated with higher rates of mental health problems. As her partner, you can't cure her PTSD, but supporting her through her treatment will help. Roll your sleeves up and get stuck in, because it will pay off, even on those days when it really doesn't feel like it.

MIKE'S STORY

During this chapter we hear from Mike, who is married to Ruth. Ruth had PTSD following the birth of their son, and we were introduced to her in Chapter 1. She came to me for treatment four years after the trauma. I'm glad to say she is recovered now, and Mike has very kindly offered to share his story of what it has been like to be the partner of someone going through birth trauma.

My name is Mike and as I start my journey into describing what it has been like to live with a loved one suffering from this condition... I am a late-middle-aged man, have a black belt in

Jujitsu, my preferred lifestyle is that of the 'rufty tufty biker'. We were married when I was at the tender age of thirty-eight (I am fourteen years Ruth's senior by the way) and I am now fifty-seven. Now Ruth's marital plumbing had always been suspect, but she was happy to go down the route of IVF and I had to follow. We had meetings and tests... an egg donor was found... an embryo was implanted... and bang on time nine months later a little boy called Thomas appeared. And I am, very much to my surprise, a doting father.

Mike and Ruth had a happy pregnancy, were planning for a natural birth, and had decided that Ruth's birth support would be her mother, rather than Mike. However, Ruth didn't get her natural birth. She had an emergency caesarean section, before her mother or Mike could get to the hospital.

Initially I never wanted to be there at the birth but now I wish I had. Ruth's mother was not there either. She was on her way to the hospital when Ruth was taken in for the caesarean section. Ruth called her mother but she got there too late. I was on my way home from work and had just arrived in Paris airport when Ruth's mother called me to tell me I was a father.

It took four long years for Ruth to get the help she needed after the birth, and during that time Mike suffered too, while he tried to help.

What's it been like for me? Hard is an understatement. Not giving up is probably one of the hardest things. How many divorces have resulted as the consequences of this condition? Who supports the partners traumatised by their loved one suffering from birth trauma PTSD?

COMMIT TO THE JOB IN HAND

In order to be able to help your partner, you need to *want* to help your partner. You might think it obvious that you want to help, but it might not be so straightforward. For example, maybe you don't really see why you should help, because you don't really understand why they can't help themselves. Or maybe you are getting impatient, and just want it to stop. Maybe you are wondering *why* your partner can't just get on with life like other parents do. Maybe you feel that they should be able to snap out of it, or use mind over matter. This chapter is for you. Mental health problems, and in particular PTSD, are not something you can 'will' your way out of. As Mike put it:

At the time neither Ruth's mother, nor I, had any idea what Ruth had been through. Would I have reacted differently while visiting at the hospital if I did know? Very probably is the answer, but when a new baby is there one tends to be a little distracted. As far as I was concerned Ruth had given birth by caesarean section like thousands of other women and the reason it took a long time to get her back to her room was she was simply recovering from it. It would be easy to say 'be positive, look what you have got, a lovely little boy and a physically healthy wife'. And, to be honest I do… But, Ruth could never see that way and it would be an insult to her to say it.

Committing to helping your partner is an important part of helping them to get better. It's not easy. Mike was at the start of a brutal learning process about how PTSD can change people, and why it is not enough to say 'be positive'. While other professionals tried to help, he was the one left with her, day in day out, 24/7. As he put it:

What I really needed to know is what to do when Ruth had an episode. I have my strategies worked out by the harsh master of failure. Professional advice would have helped. What to say

*and what not to say. When suicide is threatened and she walks
or drives away. What do I do?*

This chapter is going to try to answer some of those
questions. It's not easy, because every sufferer is different, every
form of PTSD is different, every relationship is different, and
you are different to every other partner. I am only providing
suggestions – they are not applicable to every case. You know
her, you know you, you know what happened.

Four years on, Ruth has finally received the help she needed.
She is better. I am amazed at what Mike coped with, and I hope
that he feels it was worth it, now that he has his wife back.

WHY 'PULL YOURSELF TOGETHER' DOESN'T WORK WITH TRAUMA

Understanding the nature of the beast might help you to
stay supportive. As I said at the beginning of this chapter, if
you haven't experienced PTSD yourself, it is very difficult to
understand it, given that you cannot always see the suffering.
It may be tempting to wonder why they can't control it, or pull
themselves together, or look at the positives. After all, that
is how most of us cope with bad days. We all learn to rein
our feelings in when we are children, right? She has always
managed to do so before. So why can't she now? Having some
empathy for the fact that she actually can't control it, pull
herself together or just look at the positives is an important
part of learning how you can help. Here is an example to help
illustrate why she has less control over this than we would
otherwise think:

TRY NOT TO BLINK WHEN I CLAP MY HANDS IN FRONT OF YOUR FACE

I want to give you a challenge. You are a strong-willed person,
and you have good control of your emotions, so this should be
quite easy for you. I am going to clap my hands in front of your

face, suddenly and out of the blue. But *I promise you*, I will not touch your face, or any part of you. When I do it, I do not want you to blink. If you blink, you fail. If you keep your eyes open without flinching, you win £100. Think you can do it?

You know that this will be difficult. You will blink, because blinking is automatic, it is an inbuilt reflex designed to protect your eye from damage. Sound and sudden movement will trigger it. It is not under voluntary control. Another example is a sneeze. If I were to put a load of pepper under your nose, you would sneeze. No matter how much you try to tell yourself you won't sneeze, you actually will.

Here's the thing. PTSD is the same. The 'reliving' symptoms of PTSD are an inbuilt survival mechanism and they are automatic. Anxiety, panic attacks, flashbacks, and angry outbursts are not under voluntary control. The body takes over. No amount of willpower can stop it. It feels awful. A lot worse than a blink or a sneeze, for certain. The worst part is, that while it is happening there is no logical thought process going on. Just like when we sneeze, we momentarily stop walking – when you have a flashback or an anxiety attack, you momentarily stop thinking rationally. After the sneeze, we walk again. After the panic, we think again. This is why, during a reliving episode, it won't help to try to solve it for her, or to try to reason with her. Just be there. Tell her she's safe and you love her. Know that it will pass.

Ruth's PTSD led to her having frequent angry outbursts when she felt out of control. In Mike's words:

> I would tiptoe around Ruth in the hope that I could avoid a meltdown. I'm a late-middle-aged man, my job used to be telling high-level corporate management things they never wanted to hear... easy for a hairy bottomed motorcyclist... And yet I was now terrified of what the reaction of a 5ft 4in, 43-year-old woman would be if I should accidentally put sugar in her tea.

The point is that the sufferer cannot control the symptoms when they rear up. If they could, they would. It's not easy to get our heads around that concept, but it's important, because it helps if she feels that you are trying to understand. As Mike put it:

Getting through the wall of distress to provide comfort is particularly difficult. She is in panic mode and breaking that barrier down enough for her to listen can sometimes be nigh on impossible.

When she is having a reliving symptom of PTSD (anger, anxiety, panic) do not try to fix anything. Do not try to reason with her. Just be there. Tell her she's safe and you love her. Know that it will pass.

WHEN THEY HIDE THEIR SYMPTOMS FROM YOU

One of the biggest challenges in helping someone who is suffering can be that you can't really tell that they are suffering. It is common for men and women to hide it. There are many reasons people might hide their symptoms. Maybe they think they should be grateful that they have a healthy baby. Maybe they think other parents are always happy and cope brilliantly. Maybe they think people will judge them, or take the baby from them. Maybe they are ashamed or embarrassed. Maybe they have always prided themselves on being the one who is always strong and they can't come to terms with needing help. If the partner is the one with PTSD, maybe he thinks he doesn't have a right to be distressed because he didn't have to give birth. Maybe all of these things are true. And so, they put on a smile even though inside they feel broken. They hide it.

In the case of PTSD, this can have long-term consequences,

because PTSD, by definition, does not resolve easily on its own. If you are worried about her, do something obvious: ask her about it. Ask her how she is feeling. Ask her how she feels about the birth. Ask her how much the birth bothers her. It might be that no one else has done this yet! It will be easier for her to tell you how she is feeling if she knows that you won't judge her or blame her. She is probably judging or blaming herself, which is the reason she is hiding her feelings, so she might not believe you at first when you tell her that it's okay for her to be struggling. Sometimes it's easier just to give a hug and tell her you love her.

> If you are worried about her, ask her. Ask her how she is feeling. Ask her how she feels about the birth. Ask her how much the birth bothers her. It might be that no one else has done this yet.

A PRACTICAL JOB FOR YOU

So, you've decided you want to commit to helping. You've asked her if she's okay, and she isn't. The next thing you can do is very practical. Remember that she is going to have to recover from this trauma *at the same time* as juggling being a mother, which is a 24-hour job on its own. You can help her with that by stepping up the practical help. Clean the house, tidy stuff, do the washing, get up at night with the baby (even if she is breastfeeding), feed her, cook stuff, make sandwiches, sort the shopping, tell her to go to bed and take a rest. When you take some burden off her, you give her a little more time to recover.

We know that stress inhibits the healing process by dampening the immune response and interrupting the body's ability to recover. For more details about this, see Chapter 3. Conversely, we also know that feeling loved and having the pressure taken off can help us to heal because it activates the mind and body's natural healing process. This is even more important because she has just had a baby! Think about it: even if a mother has had a beautiful birth, she still needs time and care to help her to recover, and to learn to manage the trials and tribulations and skills that come with mothering. So imagine what she needs when she's had an awful birth! Psychologically and physically, she needs time and space to recover and regroup and heal. The more opportunities for rest that you can provide for her, and the more you can help to relieve day to day burdens, the better.

I'm suggesting that you be super-helpful, kind, considerate, empathic, practical and loving. Like I said, a bit of a superhero. This is what Mike had to do. His main advice includes:

> *Have patience and lots of it. Try not to lose your temper. This definitely won't work. I say 'try' not to lose your temper as even in a normal relationship that can be difficult sometimes.*

TAKE CARE OF YOURSELF

What does every superhero need? Well, what you don't see in the cartoons is that they need to eat, sleep, and feel that they are doing a good enough job. Which brings me to my last piece of advice. Take care of yourself. It might sound glib, and you might think that your feelings don't matter as much as hers, but think again. That adage about putting your own oxygen mask on before you put someone else's on for them is absolutely true and valid. If you don't have an oxygen mask on you will faint, and then you will be useless to someone who needs you to help them with theirs. If you want to stay strong for her, you need to be strong in the first place. If you want to stay strong for her, you have to take care of yourself. Mike found that his sense of humour was one of the things he needed to protect in order to take care of himself:

A sense of humour is required just to survive this. PTSD is not funny in any way, shape or form but if you're on the receiving end of it make sure there is something out there that still makes you laugh.

Here are a few things to think about when taking care of yourself.

- Eat well.
- Rest when you can.
- Connect a little with what you need, whether that be friends, playing sports, gaming, watching TV, going for a walk.
- Find something out there that still makes you laugh (courtesy of Mike).
- Minimise any guilt that you might be feeling. This is not your fault (even if she says it is).
- Remind yourself that it will not last forever, and she will get better (thanks to Mike for that one too).

> Take care of yourself. If you want to be strong for her, you need to stay strong for both of you.

A WORD ABOUT GUILT

Guilt can be a nasty silent little nugget of slime sometimes. As a therapist, I am constantly helping clients to silence the demons of guilt and shame. Mums are constantly battling it too – it seems to come with the territory of parenthood. And it rears its ugly head with partners too. As Mike put it:

Ruth was alone when she went through a very traumatic and frightening experience. The resulting damage to Ruth's mental health has left me with great feelings of guilt and responsibility. I am her husband and was not there to protect and support her when she needed me most. I, yes me, the fat bearded bloke sat in the corner with the beer, feels guilty nearly every time Ruth has an 'episode'. It's a little like seeing a policeman when you're driving, an underlying feeling of guilt even though you have done nothing wrong, except it's much, much worse.

If you feel guilty, you're not alone. Guilt, like pain, can sometimes be seen to be adaptive, because it motivates us to try to make things better for other people. For example, we are more likely to apologise if we feel guilty. It motivates us to repair problems in relationships. But guilt can become unhelpful if it eats us up, or we can't act on it, or we can't let it go. It can be especially pernicious if we allow it to convince us that we are a bad person somehow, or have failed. This is simply unkind and untrue. If you are struggling with guilt, try to see it for what it is – an attempt to make things better – but don't let it bully you into thinking you deserve to be punished. That is not going to keep you strong, trust me. One way to help reduce the impact that guilt can have on us is to ask ourselves 'Would I judge a friend in the same way that I am judging myself?' The answer is probably no. So why be harder on yourself than you would be on them?

FEELING LIKE YOU DIDN'T DO ENOUGH AT THE BIRTH

If you are feeling guilty about something you did or did not do at the birth, then it can help to ask yourself 'What are the actual reasons why I didn't do x, y, z?' I work with a lot of partners who describe having felt helpless at the birth, and then blame themselves for not having done more to help. The point is that hospitals are not designed to facilitate the partner's presence. Ever since the 1950s, when fathers were told they couldn't be at the birth because they were a 'biological hazard' (yes, that did happen), hospitals have viewed partners as a liability, or an annoyance to be managed rather than warmly encouraged. The reason you felt helpless is because the system is designed that way. You're merely an onlooker, and if there is an obstetric situation developing, you are either ignored entirely or pushed aside. I have heard many fathers tell me that they were left in a room on their own with no idea what was happening, not knowing if or when someone might come over to explain what was going on. There are many birth preparation classes that encourage partners to speak up and ask questions during the birth, but this is to ignore the power dynamics of large institutional hospitals. It simply ain't that easy! The system is bigger than you are, and you are not to blame for not having risen up and made yourself heard. There are ways to *influence*, and that is where the birth preparation classes come in, but ultimately, the power lies with the hospital institutions. The reason you didn't speak up was because you were subtly (and maybe not so subtly) silenced or ignored. Things are changing for the better, which is good news, but in the meantime, if you are collateral damage, try not to add to the damage by blaming yourself.

So, that takes me to the end of this chapter. There are two things I haven't said which are important. Firstly, read the rest of this book too. It will help you understand what birth trauma is, how to recover from it and when to get professional help. These are all good things to know if your partner has had a traumatic birth. Secondly, encourage your partner to get some professional help. This is especially so if she is still struggling with what happened at the birth more than three months later. (If it is only three weeks after the birth, there is every chance that she will get better spontaneously, especially with some help and support from you, but it's still good to have some options up your sleeve in case things don't improve). And if you get help, but it doesn't seem to be helping, then don't give up. Try some other help. There are options out there, different professionals within and outside of the NHS, and some good professionals and some not so good, and some that aren't a good fit for your partner, and some that are. Ruth went through general practitioners and psychiatrists and diagnoses of bipolar disorder and various medications before finding the help that was right for her. She and Mike persisted, and in the end she was finally on the road to recovery after four long years.

> Get some professional help. If at first the help doesn't help, try some other help. Don't give up.

Finally, I'll leave you with one quote that illustrates how lonely it can be to be supporting someone suffering from PTSD. In Mike's own words:

What did I need? A cuddle would have been nice...

– 6 –

IT'S NOT JUST BIRTH TRAUMA: OTHER AREAS OF PERINATAL TRAUMA

Trigger warning: contains vivid details of distressing scenarios which you may find distressing. Please take care of yourself.

I have been working with perinatal trauma for many years, and it has become apparent that it's not just birth trauma that I am seeing in the perinatal period. I work with PTSD, but I also work with trauma that doesn't quite meet the criteria for PTSD but nonetheless responds really well to trauma-focused therapy. I think this is because the mechanism is the same – the amygdala has captured the memory, and has not allowed the memory to be processed in the neocortex, which creates a stress reaction every time the memory surfaces, for whatever reason. This chapter looks at other ways in which trauma can manifest during the perinatal period.

TRAUMA DUE TO BABY IN SPECIAL CARE

If your baby was born prematurely and spent time in neonatal intensive care (NICU), then your mental health will have been tested. The rates of PTSD in parents of premature babies are thought to be as high as 16% – a lot higher than the 2–5% for birth trauma (BLISS, 2018). Rates of anxiety and depression are also higher for parents of NICU babies. And yet most parents are sent home with their babies, expecting a fairytale happy ending. They are not asked about their mental health. They are not screened for PTSD. NICU wards are not the most comforting of places: they are full of bright lights, cold plastic and equipment, loud shrill beeping sounds, and babies who are sick and might die. Including your own.

On top of that, you might have to witness your baby be subjected to painful intervention, left alone, and feel the fear that he or she might not make it. It seems obvious that this is going to be a source of PTSD, and yet this has only just begun to be recognised by the service. Many parts of the country are investing in mental health support for parents, and there is recognition that this support needs to be available long after the baby has been brought home, because the symptoms of PTSD will not necessarily manifest until a few months after the homecoming. If you are suffering from the traumatic effects of having had a baby in NICU, then know that it is okay to not be okay. It is okay to be suffering now, even if you are grateful that your baby is fine. It is okay to ask for help.

I'm hoping that this book will help validate your feelings, and that once you are at home with a baby who is safe, you can begin to think about your needs too. It's time to build yourself back up again so that you can move forward in your parenting journey, free of the possible effects of trauma. Your nerves have been frazzled, you have been scared and tired, and your nervous system will need time to resettle and heal. It is likely that there will be things that trigger your anxiety, in line with what scared you the most. For example, you may well really struggle whenever your baby is unwell. Although you know logically that it is just a cold, your amygdala is likely to fire off, and your anxiety will be triggered. Or you may find that you struggle to respond to your baby when she cries – you know logically how to respond, but emotionally you feel paralysed when she cries. Or you may find that you can't bear to watch him have injections. The list goes on. If these reactions go on for months, therapy for trauma can help.

BREASTFEEDING TRAUMA

It is only just becoming understood that women are being traumatised by their experiences of trying to breastfeed their babies. This may be because it has been assumed that breastfeeding your baby is not a life or death situation. However, experience tells us that it certainly can feel that way for many mothers. Of course, in our evolutionary past, it could have been a life or death situation, because if a baby wouldn't feed, that would suggest they were ill (I am presuming that babies and mothers didn't need to learn to breastfeed like we do now, because it would have been something that girls witnessed throughout their childhood, and if there were any latch issues, the baby would be wet-nursed by a relative or friend).

When there is blood and damage to your nipples involved, it can seem life-threatening. When there is tremendous grief involved at not being able to do what you passionately want to do, it can seem devastating. And when you are in a society that has so many negative and mixed messages about infant feeding, which has such misguided and damaging practices around feeding, such as blaming women, disregarding the importance of this for some women, focusing on what is 'best' for baby rather than taking the mother's needs and wishes into account, failing to prioritise proper breastfeeding support and training, failing to crack down on formula industries while simultaneously criticising formula feeding parents... the list goes on. For a deeper understanding of the political and cultural issues around infant feeding, see Gabrielle Palmer's *Why the Politics of Breastfeeding Matters* (Pinter & Martin, 2016).

Breastfeeding trauma is only recently being recognised as

a cause for concern, and is, once again, associated with a lack of support. Professor Amy Brown's research, during which she interviewed and listened to many women who describe feeling traumatised while breastfeeding, gives us accounts from mothers. They describe feelings of horror, helplessness, fear, lack of support associated with being unable to breastfeed when they wanted to be able to do so, and many of their reactions are in line with a diagnosis of PTSD. One woman talks about flashbacks:

If I hear about another mum talking about how much she struggled, I get flashbacks to those hideous, guilt wrenched days even though she's five years old now.

Another describes how she avoids things related to breastfeeding:

I can't read anything about breastfeeding or babies in general. It's too traumatic still. I am a bit better now but went through a phase where I even needed to avoid the baby aisle in the supermarket as it would trigger how I felt or put me on edge for the rest of the day without realising why.

Breastfeeding trauma, just like birth trauma, can activate a sense of shame, as illustrated by the mother who said '*I hate myself and think I am not a good enough mother. Nothing anyone says or does can change the fact I failed*'. The sense of not being able to move on from it is felt by this woman, who said '*I find myself getting preoccupied with babies and breastfeeding long after I read an article. It plays on my mind and goes round and round and I find it difficult to concentrate.*' I'm sorry if you have experienced this first-hand. You are certainly not alone. The trauma can be over a blurred period of time, rather than one specific event, but it still counts as trauma. There will probably be 'hotspots', or specific moments of horror or misery that you remember, and it is these that a trauma therapist would work on with you. Even if the traumatic period is over now, and things are fine, it may continue to affect how you feel about your mothering, or your relationship with your baby. It may affect you again if you move on to have another baby. Either way, be aware that you could be suffering from trauma symptoms, and that some self-care in the form of acknowledging this and deciding to get some help could be a great way forward.

TRAUMA IN FATHERS AND PARTNERS

It took a long time to raise awareness of PTSD in mothers, but even longer to recognise that PTSD in birth partners is also something that needs attention. Fathers are expected to be in the delivery room, but are rarely prepared for what they might encounter. When I was a trainee hypnobirthing instructor, I was at a training day when the instructor (the wonderful midwife Mary Cronk) checked with us that we had seen a baby being born before showing us photos of crowning babies. She told us that she forgets so easily that when you aren't used to seeing babies be born, it can come as a bit of a shock to see the full works in action.

I suddenly realised that we don't ask partners this before enthusiastically presuming that they are happy to be at the birth, and encouraging them to take a look as the baby comes out. We don't even ask them how they feel about being at the birth in the first place. I have heard from many fathers who say that they are scared to be at the birth – they worry they will faint with the blood, they worry that they will see something they can't get out of their minds, they worry that they will fail to support her, or feel like a spare part. Tokophobia (morbid fear of childbirth) can affect men too. But if a man says that he is frightened to be at the birth, he will be dismissed, laughed at or criticised. It is presumed that he will be there. Partners are provided with almost no preparation or emotional support for being at the birth. On the contrary, they are often expected to be the emotional support or to communicate the birth plan, in order to be useful.

The kinds of things that I have seen with fathers who have been traumatised stem from a pre-morbid belief that birth is inherently dangerous. This can mean that when they see medical equipment or intervention, they get scared that their partner or their baby is going to die. And, if you remember from Chapter 3, having experienced an event in which you thought you, or someone else, was going to die or be harmed is the first criterion for a diagnosis of PTSD. I have worked with fathers who were traumatised when the staff said that the mother needed an 'emergency caesarean'. They didn't realise that it wasn't an emergency as such, it was more like an 'unscheduled caesarean' (as the vast majority of unplanned caesarean sections are). Another father I worked with was traumatised when he heard that his baby was just going on the 'resuscitation' bed. He didn't know that this happens to 10% of new babies, and is not a sign that the baby is about to die.

The language used in hospitals manages to alienate and frighten a lot of parents, as do the uniforms, medical equipment and so on. Furthermore, I have heard many fathers tell me that they felt abandoned, because their partner was whisked away for a procedure and they were left in a hospital room, alone, and with just their imagination to keep them company. More research and awareness-raising around this issue is needed. In my experience, the issues are the same as they are for women that birth. Proper communication and emotional support from the birth professionals could prevent a lot of PTSD in partners. The issues that partners who have been traumatised are faced with are, in my experience, similar to the issues that birthing mothers experience: they are left with traumatic memories of the time that they thought their partner was dying, and consequent feelings of guilt and shame about what they did or didn't do, feeling out of control, unheard, and feelings of having failed. Furthermore, they too hide their suffering, but maybe for different reasons. As one father put it 'I never would of brought it up to anyone, even my wife: how could I possibly tell her how traumatised I was when she's the person that had the ordeal of having a baby' (Daniels et al).

Recovery from trauma often involves helping partners to see that they were disempowered in a system that unwittingly disregards their presence, their feelings and their emotional welfare. It was not their fault. This can be complicated by the fact that some mothers also blame their partner, because they think that he or she should have spoken up, or protected her, or been firmer about declining intervention, or insisted on intervention and so forth. Not being listened to came up as a theme in one research study of fathers' experiences of traumatic births, as described by one father who said 'I felt mostly like a spare wheel to be kept out of the way'. Another father described 'being made to feel like the enemy, a useless caveman that has thoughtlessly impregnated this innocent girl' (Daniels et al). And I see the broken parents who blame themselves and each other for the fact that the birth was traumatic.

This is part of the fallacy that hospitals 'share' their power, and are interested in listening to birth preferences, and that the birth partner can be the advocate for the mother. As a birth doula, I see time and time again how incredibly difficult this job is for birth partners when they are on hospital turf, unsure in the face of uniformed staff who flippantly disregard him because they are busy. And the tragedy is that they then feel unable to ask for, or get, the help that they might need to heal from their birth trauma. If you are a birth partner and you feel that you were traumatised from the birth, then don't disregard that. There are some very effective therapies out there that can help you to move on. If you feel that your partner was traumatised but they are not ready to acknowledge that, then know that that is not unusual. We talk about it being difficult for birth mothers to admit that they are struggling. It is, in my opinion, even harder for the partners, because society does not think that birth is about them, and because men are supposed to be strong and support their partners.

POSTNATAL WARD TRAUMA

We have known for a while that women can become traumatised during birth. We know that being treated with kindness and compassion can mitigate against the chances of developing trauma symptoms. What is less well known is that women can become traumatised on the postnatal ward following the birth of their baby too. I know this because I see it in my work. For years I have been working with women who have been traumatised in those first 24 hours after birth. I think there is a vulnerability in new mothers that is not recognised or understood in our culture. We know about the importance of attachment, bonding and breastfeeding for the health of the nation as a whole (not necessarily for individuals). We know that the leading cause of maternal death associated with having babies during the first year after birth, is maternal suicide (MBRRACE-UK). We know that babies on the whole, statistically speaking, thrive better when they have calmer people around them.

Any compassionate culture that really understands these issues would take care of new mothers. New parents are holding future generations' welfare in their hands. Let's help them on their journey. Let's cherish new mothers, wrap them up in warm blankets, feed them homemade soup, tell them they are amazing, and give them practical and emotional support as they recover from birth. Let's help them feel empowered as mothers, rather than broken. Let's give them privacy and peace in the first few days of their lives as new mothers. Other societies do this, so why can't we?

Consider what we are doing instead. How many new mothers do you know who would say they loved the postnatal ward? How many hospitals make the postnatal ward homely and welcoming? They put money into birthing pools with dim lights because they know the importance of oxytocin for physiological birth, and the need to reduce stress hormones during labour. However, oxytocin is just as important for bonding and breastfeeding. We need the same attention paid to postnatal wards as there is for birth rooms, in order to avoid trauma and distress in those wards. We need to value the care that midwives provide postnatally, and not reduce their numbers so dramatically that they are also burned out, exhausted and desperate. In some wards, the treatment that new mothers receive is the antithesis of compassionate care. Lucy's story is a sad reflection of that. She told me of her experience on the postnatal ward. I share it here, despite the fact that it makes sad reading, and is difficult to comprehend. But I hear it all the time. I guess I want to share these stories to give other people the courage to share their own experiences, and not to dismiss their own reality of what has happened to them.

LUCY'S STORY

I introduced you to Lucy on page 95. I described her as a grounded, rational, emotionally intelligent and confident person. I'm not just saying that to be nice. She really was, in my opinion, psychologically healthy. Her psychological health was put to the test when she had a medically complicated pregnancy, which culminated in a mismanaged birth, ending up in an emergency caesarean section with a general anaesthetic, no pain relief upon waking from the operation, and a hospital that proceeded to 'lose' her case notes. I have spared some other details. Suffice it to say, it was a challenge.

Now, if that had happened to anyone that you know and vaguely care about, and you were there to support her, what would you suggest for her? Fill your boots. How are we going to help Lucy to recover from this awful experience? I would guess that most of us would think of the same things. She'll need some time in hospital. She'll need rest. She'll need pain medication. She'll benefit from sensitivity to what she's been through, and time with her loved ones. Good old-fashioned tender loving care and attention. Lucy did receive this when she was in the recovery room, in the time between the surgery and going up to the postnatal ward. She had been cared for, reassured that all was well, cuddled her baby, breastfed him, left in peace with her baby, her husband and one kind midwife. However, when she got to the postnatal ward, things changed.

In her words 'it was a horrible place, we were all cramped in, the staff were horrible witches – stern and shouting… cruel'. She told me that the staff were rude, dismissive, and ignored her medical needs, never mind her psychological ones. This was in a normal London hospital! She was vomiting every hour, getting dehydrated, and when she asked for fluids, they ignored her. She had to insist loudly that she needed fluids. She was there for two days before she escaped. In that time, someone said to her 'Please do not talk to me while I'm doing the medication'. The experience became so unpleasant for Lucy, that, in her own words, 'I went into a dark, scared place… I felt like they were torturing me, abusing me'. When this developed into a panic attack, she heard the staff say, from behind the curtain, 'She's really making a fuss'.

On the second day Lucy 'lost it'. She became angry and hysterical, shouting and screaming at them. She felt utterly trapped. After the second day, she and her husband planned their escape. They hid the fact that she was still vomiting (by literally hiding the vomit), and they pretended that she had had a wee, when she hadn't (she actually faked it). Although she could have discharged herself against medical advice, she did not feel safe enough to do so, and neither did her husband. They literally thought that their baby might be taken from them if they did that. That is how unsafe they felt.

Given Lucy's story, it's easy to see that problems on the postnatal ward, or when baby is in special care, can also lead to traumatic memories. Lucy needed to lift the trauma of the birth as well as the postnatal ward. I often work with women who have no birth trauma – but they then become traumatised by their postnatal ward experience. It's a time when other cultures nurture and look after their new mothers, insisting that they rest well, eat well, and be looked after. Our postnatal wards do not do that. And I think that puts lives at risk.

FOURTH TRIMESTER TRAUMA

Sometimes, trauma can develop in the first six weeks postnatally, if the baby isn't settled, and is crying inconsolably, but the mother's concerns aren't taken seriously, or she feels helpless, distressed, isolated and worried for her baby. Did you know that the sound of a crying baby raises mothers' cortisol levels dramatically? This makes sense really. We've evolved to respond to our baby's cry. Frankly, being alone with a very distressed baby, night after night, feeling helpless, hopeless and desperate, can lay down traumatic memories that stay with you. I have often heard this given as a reason why people are not able to consider having another baby, even though they had originally wanted more. I do not think mothers were designed to spend any time alone with babies. In our evolutionary past there would have been a village of caring, older, wiser women around to relieve our distress and help us through. Without that support, our mental health is put to the test. Fathers or partners might try to help, but they are not necessarily wiser or more experienced with babies, and they also have their own worries and concerns to deal with. Trauma doesn't have to be associated with just one memory: it can be associated with multiple events that bleed into each other, creating a traumatic time period, rather than a single traumatic event. If this is relevant to you, and you feel that deep down you would like another baby, but you are terrified of going through the same thing again, then know that therapy to relieve the trauma symptoms can really help.

TRAUMA IN BABIES

Can babies be traumatised? That is a question I often ask midwives at my workshops. There is always some level of disagreement in the room. Some think 'Of course babies get traumatised', while others think 'Of course they don't'. Some look at me blankly because it's never occurred to them to consider it before. Have a little think, and ask yourself how you would answer the question. Do they or don't they? The way that we view babies has changed dramatically over recent years, and continues to do so. We used to call babies 'it', and we used to regard them as things, rather than sentient little beings experiencing the world in their own way. We used to think they couldn't even feel pain. Not so long ago, psychologists were saying that babies didn't have the brain capacity to be able to register pain. It was believed that what looked like a reaction to pain was 'just' a reflex (I know! It's hard to believe). Nowadays, when I ask a room of midwives whether babies can feel pain, they all emphatically say 'Yes, of course they can feel pain'. If I ask the question 'Can babies remember?' most say yes (but not all). But when I ask 'Can babies be traumatised?' I get a mixed response. We may have moved towards knowing that babies feel pain, and believing that they remember, but the jury is still out on whether they can be traumatised. I'm not a soothsayer, but I do believe that in a decade or so it will seem obvious to everyone that babies can be traumatised, and that we should take notice of this, pay good attention to it, and do something about it.

MARIA'S STORY

When Maria, a hypnobirthing client of mine, had her first baby, she had him at home in her peaceful calm room, in the birth pool that had been especially set up. Her husband and two midwives were in attendance. When a baby is born in water, the way in which a baby 'wakes up' or transitions to lung breathing is slightly different to what midwives usually see, which is a crying stressed baby who has just had his oxygen supply severed by the cutting of the cord. But because Maria's baby had the cord intact, and because baby was peaceful, not crying etc., the midwives chose to be extra certain, and they decided to cut the cord, take baby out of the water, put him on a towel at the side, and get him breathing and crying nice and quickly. He was then given back to Maria, who had stepped out of the pool onto a sofa by the side. When Maria told me her birth story, not much thought was given to this little hiccup. It had been a pretty great birth, all things considered, and everyone was thrilled.

However, at my postnatal visit, Maria and her husband raised one issue that had been bothering them slightly. They told me that their baby was calm, serene, slept well, and had all the hallmarks of a very contented little lad. Except for when he had a bath. They told me he cried dramatically and inconsolably, every time they bathed him, much to the distress of everyone involved. After the bath, he was fine again. I asked for more detail, which they gave. 'Well, it's when we take him out of the bath, and put him on the towel'. I asked how they do that. 'We put him on his back, onto a towel that is already laid out for him'.

As they said the words, we all made the connection. Their little boy was reliving the trauma of the midwives' intervention, each and every time he was taken out of warm water and laid flat out on a towel on his back. His amygdala was reacting, with a kind of flashback every time. Following our conversation, his parents changed how they took him out of the bath. Instead of lying him on his back, they would have the towel ready in the crook of their body, and they would snuggle him upright, into their stomach, into the *towel and roll him up into their body. And he stopped hating baths immediately.*

In this case, it was easy to see the connection between a traumatic experience and the anxious reaction, because the baby was well in all other areas of his life and he was generally relaxed. He didn't have PTSD; he had a specific trauma reaction (situational anxiety, described in the section on triggers in Chapter 3). But what if some babies experience trauma that is not so discreet, trauma that is more pronounced, or more pervasive? Think about those babies that society likes to describe as 'difficult', or, even worse, not a 'good' baby. These ways of describing distressed babies tell us quite a lot about our ongoing attitudes towards babies. We don't see their distress. Maybe the baby startles easily, or wakes up scared a lot, or has indigestion associated with stress, or has trouble sleeping, or cries a lot, or can't be settled very easily, or sleeps for only 20 minutes at a time, and so on. These could all be 'symptoms' of PTSD. But because our society has yet to come round to the idea that babies are sentient human beings, capable of mental health problems, we are arguably missing the symptoms of PTSD in babies.

If you think your baby may be showing signs of trauma or distress from a difficult birth, I know that this might be distressing for you. Please be reassured that it was not your fault. Often parents feel that their baby is damaged, which can be so upsetting for parents. But this is just a temporary thing, just as a bruise caused by some kind of accident would be temporary. Babies heal from bruises, and they heal from difficult births. Their brains are 'plastic', which means that they change and grow and adapt very quickly and easily (much more quickly and effectively than an adult's brain). All the ideas in this book about how to heal also apply to your baby. The things that will help your baby recover include a calm, peaceful, loving environment, which will serve to activate the relaxation system, and deactivate the stress system. Your loving connection will help your baby to recover, even when you can't tell that your presence is helping. Did you know that when a baby cries in your arms, they produce fewer stress hormones than when they cry in a cot? Our brains are designed to heal, and that includes your baby's brain. Give your baby the conditions for good healing which are discussed in Chapter 4, and he or she will be on the path to recovery.

TRAUMA AND PERINATAL OCD

When Katie's baby was eight weeks old, Katie was suddenly struck by an anxiety so bad, out of the blue, that she very quickly sought help from her GP. She was tearful and distressed. Her GP diagnosed postnatal depression with anxiety. She had been experiencing very bad anxiety, panic attacks and what she described as 'paranoia' for about two weeks when I saw her. She told me that it had come on after she stopped breastfeeding. Could there be a connection?

Katie explained: 'I feel out of control, I'm a BIG control freak, and I usually have lots of energy and get loads done, but at the moment, I feel that I have hardly any energy, I feel so scared, I don't know what's wrong with me'. She had also lost her beloved grandmother in the past few weeks. Katie was very tearful during this session, and I could see why her GP thought she was going into postnatal depression. It would have been tempting to think 'big control freak, gets completely thrown by a new baby, can't control anything, and develops postnatal depression as a result'.

But I asked Katie a question which took us down another path. I asked 'What are you most afraid of?' She replied 'getting psychosis and wanting to kill my baby'. She said 'I panic about it every day. I worry that if I have these negative thoughts, I might end up believing them, and they might become real'. She continued: 'I feel so sad about this, I get scared that I'll drop him, so I hold him tight instead and tell myself that I AM a good mummy'.

It became obvious that Katie was suffering from something called perinatal or maternal obsessional compulsive disorder. This is a very common anxiety disorder associated with having a baby, but is not often diagnosed or well understood among professionals.

But what has this story got to do with birth trauma? Well, what is also not well understood among mental health professionals is that OCD is very often brought on by, or associated with, a traumatic experience. It would seem that the traumatic experience can lead to the brain being over-sensitised to a specific fear or scenario, and that the brain then cannot stop thinking about this repeating fearful scenario, experiencing ongoing intrusions. So, what was Katie's traumatic experience that led to the development of perinatal OCD? Well, it turns out there were two.

Katie's intrusions were concerned with two themes. The first was 'I'm going to drop my baby'. While this is a very common theme in maternal OCD, Katie's thought was rather more specific. During therapy, Katie became aware that all her intrusions were about *damage to his head*. We worked out that this was associated with the horror of seeing her baby's poor little bruised head after he was born. The memories of his damaged head had become traumatically held within her mind. She had then gone on to re-experience his bruised head in the form of intrusions, which horrified her. Because they horrified her, she tried to push them away. But they kept coming back. And horrifying her even more, and leading her to believe that she was a bad mother capable of dropping her baby.

The second theme was associated with 'I'm going to go into a psychotic breakdown and end up killing myself and my baby'. This rather dramatic fear had become established during one very stressful night in hospital. Katie's baby had been successfully treated for sepsis. This rather scary period of her baby being unwell had ended with a night in hospital with just Katie and the baby. Katie's husband had not been allowed to stay, as only one adult was permitted. I'm not sure why this is a rule. But it's often the case that hospitals have policies that don't always seem necessary. So Katie had to stay on her own, in a room with no other adult, and her baby who had been very ill but was now safe in recovery. No one had checked whether Katie was okay, or how she felt. She didn't think to check this for herself either (we can trust mothers to take care of their babies, but they are notoriously poor at taking care of themselves!).

So, as the awful night unfolded, Katie was in a hospital room, on her own, upset, tired, very anxious from the fact that she had had a very scary time while her baby had been treated for sepsis, unable to sleep, getting more and more tired, more and more distressed, but unable to settle herself or calm herself, and having no one else around to help her either. Her thoughts took hold, and she felt like she was going mad. She was terrified at that prospect, so she tried to push the thoughts out of her mind, but it just got worse and worse. By the time she got home, she had got into a vicious cycle of being obsessed with the thought that she might go mad and kill her baby – a thought that had originally been planted while reading a very graphic and tragic account of postnatal psychosis. Be careful what you read! What she didn't know was that postnatal psychosis and postnatal anxiety are very different kettles of fish. In the former, there is indeed some danger of the mother hurting herself and her baby. In the latter, there is not the same danger: although it can feel pretty awful, it is not considered dangerous. In fact, maternal OCD is often seen in the most loving and diligent of mothers, and for this reason professionals do not worry about the baby when a mother is diagnosed with it.

Because Katie got to therapy quickly, she managed to feel much better after six sessions of cognitive behavioural therapy which focused on the trauma using the rewind method. After therapy, Katie described feeling normal again, able to enjoy her baby again, and being back to her old self. Of course, she can never be quite back to her old self, because she is now a mother! But negotiating that journey is so much easier when trauma has been taken out of the equation.

A BRIEF EXPLANATION OF MATERNAL OCD

Maternal OCD is an anxiety disorder that develops about pregnancy and birth. The anxiety concerns the fear that your baby will be harmed, and that you, as the mother, are responsible for keeping the baby safe. Obsessions involve uninvited and unwanted scary thoughts that something bad will happen, or that you, as a mother, will do something bad or neglectful. When these horrible thoughts enter your head, you are horrified, terrified, ashamed, aghast. Almost like a mini trauma reaction, your brain goes into a shock reaction. You try to push the thoughts or images away because they are so awful. But that doesn't work. (After all, if I told you to push away the image of an elephant in a tutu dancing on a stage, would that work? No. You see an elephant in a tutu no matter how hard you try not to. And the more you try, the harder it gets).

When pushing the thoughts away doesn't work, you develop other ways to reassure yourself, like an antidote to the terrifying thought or image. This might be things you do or things that you think (such as repeat hand washing, asking your partner to bath your baby, not letting anyone else hold your baby, holding your baby tighter, checking that your mum thinks you're a good mum, counting to five and so on). These things that you do to help yourself feel better may be obviously related to the scary thought, or seem a bit more random, but the point is that you feel temporarily better, so you get hooked on doing it every time the bad thought or image comes up. The bad thoughts keep coming, so you furiously keep doing the thing that temporarily helps, and you get into a vicious cycle. It's awful being stuck in this vicious cycle: your anxiety is climbing and climbing because you are having to tolerate these awful images and thoughts that you actually believe may happen, or you actually believe make you a bad mum. Because of the shame associated with the belief that you might harm your baby, people are scared to mention it to others, because they think it means they are a bad mother, because they believe that to think 'I'm going to hurt my baby' means that they are indeed going to hurt their baby.

Let me reassure you. These thoughts *don't* mean that you are going to hurt your baby. And they *don't* mean that you are a bad mum. Quite the opposite! It is because you are a diligent, responsible and caring mum, that the thoughts are so odious to you. The link between maternal OCD and trauma is that OCD often has a cause that goes back to a specific traumatic experience or memory. This includes stories that you might have heard – it doesn't need to have happened directly to you.

BIRTH TRAUMA AS A GRIEF REACTION

Birth trauma often encompasses a sense of grief. We often think about grief as being something that happens when someone we care about dies. But we can experience a grief reaction when we lose things other than people. We can experience grief when we lose a dream. Or an expectation. When you've been through a bad birth, there were expectations and dreams you had which didn't happen. This can lead to a grief reaction. Grief that you didn't get the birth you were hoping for, or you didn't get the skin-to-skin that you were looking forward to, or you didn't feel a rush of love for your baby, or didn't get to breastfeed your baby.

Now, before I go on, I just want to clear up a common misconception. I think midwives and birth professionals are very aware of the fact that women often feel devastated when their hopes of a fulfilling birth are dashed. I often hear people say that women shouldn't 'set themselves up' for disappointment by preparing for, and hoping for, wonderful births. This gets my goat a little. Firstly, it's a way of blaming the mother for being upset about her birth. But secondly, I think that to say that women should not expect too much of birth is a little like saying 'don't expect sex to be nice, expect it to be brutal and violent and dangerous so that you're not disappointed'. Women have the right to expect sex to be consensual and non-violent. Shouldn't that be the case for birth too? Believing that birth might be joyful and empowering is something every woman should be allowed to do, just as she is allowed to believe that her first sexual contact might be pleasurable and loving. If you are feeling bereft because you didn't get the birth you were hoping for, then you have every right to feel grief for that loss.

It's important to honour your grief, rather than belittle it or ignore it, because then it can heal. Our brains and bodies have an inbuilt way of processing and working through grief. Grief is normal. Grief can't be avoided, just like we can't avoid a snotty nose when our bodies are recovering from a cold. The five stages of grieving that many psychological therapists use to understand the healing process, apply to birth too. The stages include shock, denial, searching, anger, bargaining and acceptance. The idea is that we can move through the stages in different ways, at different speeds, sometimes missing some altogether, sometimes coming back to a previous one. The general consensus among therapists is that the aim is to reach acceptance at some point in your life. Healing grief is a journey. It hurts. And we can never really get over what happened, or stop hurting, but we can come to a place of peace. However, while we are navigating that journey, we can get 'stuck' at certain stages, which prevents us from reaching a place of acceptance. This is the time that we might suggest professional help to reignite the normal process of moving through the stages.

Let's take a look at each of these stages:

THE SHOCK PHASE is probably common after any birth, even if you've had a straightforward birth! Feeling bewildered, overwhelmed, speechless, or disbelief about what just happened is common. If you had a traumatic birth, the sense of shock can be profound. It can lead to a sense of paralysis, both emotionally and physically. When the shock stage doesn't lift, we might find ourselves feeling constantly in a dream-like state, or not really 'with it', or dissociating a lot, or numb to feelings and events.

THE DENIAL STAGE is the part where you might try to move on super quickly, and deny that it matters, or that it has any consequence for you. You might find yourself saying 'Oh, it's okay, at least I have a healthy baby. I'm okay, I'm going to put my past behind me and get on with my future. The birth doesn't matter'. Denial is regarded as a form of coping, so that we can come to terms with everything at a gentler pace, rather than being faced with the true magnitude of the loss all at once. Your brain is looking after you, even if you're not aware of it.

THE BARGAINING STAGE represents an attempt to make sense of what happened, and to try to get some sense of control back. It can show itself in terms of ruminating about how things could have been different, with thoughts such as 'Where did I go wrong, if only I hadn't done this, that, or the other... I shouldn't have allowed that obstetrician in the room, I should have shouted louder, I should have had a home birth,' and so on. It can also involve trying to find a way to make it better: 'Next time I'll hire a doula, next time I'll write a birth plan' and so on.

THE ANGER STAGE represents an acknowledgement that what happened to you was wrong (even if it was just bad luck – it can still feel incredibly unfair) and it is nature's way of ramping up your energy levels to do something about the problem. You might find yourself warning other people never to have a baby, you might find yourself writing to the hospital, or considering legal action, or blaming your partner, or resenting your baby for causing all this. Mostly, anger is a form of dissipating energy, and can feel quite cathartic. If, however, you feel that you are stuck in your anger, in that you never seem to be able to move on, or that it is creating problems in your life, because you are constantly feeling it, or it is exploding at the wrong times, or it is being targeted at the wrong people (such as your baby), then it might be an idea to seek some outside help to shift you on from this stuck anger.

THE DEPRESSION STAGE is where you feel really sad that it happened, you feel listless, you don't eat well or sleep well, and you want to cry a lot. This is the opposite of the anger phase – nature is not wanting you to ramp up your energy. She wants you to shut down and rest for a bit. Depression drains us of motivation and energy; it deactivates us. This is tough if you are looking after a new baby, in a society which believes you should just carry on as normal. There is a theory that the function of depression is to motivate other people to rally round and look after us. Unfortunately, that doesn't happen so easily now that we live within our own four walls, and we pretend we are okay when we are not, and people are too busy with their own lives to have time to cook for you, visit you, take care of you and so on. When depression is a function of grief and loss for the birth you didn't have, you should find that this phase doesn't last too long. Again, as with the anger, if you find it dragging on, or it leaves you struggling to cope, it's probably time to get some help.

THE ACCEPTANCE STAGE is where we can come to terms with what happened, and move on emotionally from it. The memory is always there, but the pain associated with it feels more peaceful, more settled, and more in the past. This is more likely to happen when we have grasped that it wasn't our fault, that it was bad luck, that there may have been a reason why it happened (if you have some spiritual beliefs, in particular, or believe in fate). Acceptance often also comes with the ability to see what we couldn't see before: that there are some lessons that can be learned from what happened, or some good that can be gleaned from it. It can be really hard to find any lessons learned, and that is what therapy often helps us to do.

TRAUMA IN BIRTH PROFESSIONALS

Midwives get traumatised too. Research suggests that between 17 and 33% of midwives experience PTSD during the course of their professional life (Paterson). In a system which can be accused of being overly medicalised, patriarchal, misogynistic and racist, of disregarding women's and babies' experiences, of reigniting past experiences of sexual abuse, and of ignoring the voices and wishes of birthing women, midwives are victims too. Many midwives go into the profession with a natural respect for birth and birthing women, and they look to support and nurture women as they birth, gaining a sense of empowerment and satisfaction from deep relationships with the women that they serve. As such, they are vulnerable to being traumatised by witnessing the mother being mistreated. Jenny Paterson has studied trauma in midwives, and she writes:

> Around 70% of midwives witness poor, disrespectful, or indifferent interpersonal care of women or high levels of obstetric interventions. Witnessing women's trauma leaves midwives feeling horror (intense feeling of fear, shock and disgust) and guilt.

Another aspect of trauma for midwives concerns the levels of abuse that they experience directly, in a system which undermines them, undervalues them and is overly punitive. I say that if midwives were mainly men, they would not be paid what they are paid, their supervisory system would be less punitive, they would have more resources to do their job properly, and the 'soft' skills of compassion, intuition, connection and empathy which are so important for good midwifery, for reducing trauma and for saving lives, would be recognised, valued, and rewarded. In the words of one midwife:

I am a midwife with eight years' experience and I am tired. I am tired of the punitive practice, the fear, the paperwork, the audits, the inspections and the nights on the sofa sobbing after another dreadful shift. I am tired of the negativity, the bullying that I see young midwives subjected to and the absolute inability of individuals to freely give outstanding care to women. In the wake of Francis and Kirkup we see ourselves lambasted in the press and vilified by the media. We are trying so hard as a profession to change and to give one another the courage to question the entrenched practice we see every day – but one or two midwives in each trust is not enough. We must all come together as women and declare that it is time to focus not on midwife-led care but woman-centred care. We have a long road ahead of us. (Anonymous author, *The Guardian*, 2015)

It's not just midwives. Secondary trauma, or vicarious trauma, is the process of being traumatised by witnessing traumatic situations – you don't need to be the one at risk in order to get PTSD. Other birth professionals, such as midwifery care assistants, birth doulas and doctors can be traumatised too. The research on that is more scarce, however. If you are a midwife or healthcare professional and you think you have experienced PTSD, then you probably have. You might find that you are avoiding certain aspects of your job, or that just going into work is becoming more and more difficult. It is a hazard of your job – it is not a weakness of your personality. Prioritise your self-care and get some help for it. We lose many midwives due to them leaving the profession, and the tragedy is that we tend to lose some of the most compassionate and empathic ones – in other words, some of the best ones. There are plenty of therapists out there to help you if you don't want to leave your job, or if you think that your fear might be affecting your work. Don't keep quiet about this – it is the workplace that is the problem here, not you. We need to talk about this. Maternity care needs to take care of its professionals within a compassionate workplace, in order to reduce trauma and the ripple effects that trauma leaves behind.

WHEN YOU HAVEN'T EVEN GOT A HEALTHY BABY

The fact that some babies die is something which touches us deeply at a human level, but we never think it will happen to us. If it has happened to you, you will need to walk the relentless and brutal path of grief. Your loss is almost unbearable on its own, and for that reason, you do not need the added burden of PTSD in your struggles. Losing your baby is a traumatic experience in and of itself, and it is natural to feel shocked and horrified and angry and anxious. However, if, after a number of months, you are experiencing flashbacks, nightmares, marked anxiety or anger, and are avoiding reminders of the traumatic memory to the detriment of your recovery, then it might be that you have some trauma symptoms to contend with along with the grief process.

If there are specific 'hot spots' in your memory, moments which you cannot bear to remember, then that is a sign that you are dealing with trauma symptoms as well as grief. Grief is a normal reaction to loss, and as such, can't be 'treated' or fixed. It has to be experienced, as part of the recovery journey. However, trauma symptoms which are not resolving can inhibit recovery, weakening your resilience when you most need it in order to move through your grief. Therapy can help you heal the trauma so that you can focus better on moving through the grief. Take a look at Chapter 8, on possible therapies that are out there to help you.

– 7 –

HOW TRAUMA CAN AFFECT OTHER AREAS OF YOUR LIFE

RELATIONSHIP STRAIN

Learning to navigate our relationship when a new baby arrives is a challenge for any couple with a new baby. How to support each other, how to take care of ourselves while we do so, knowing how to manage everyday stresses, navigating the sharing of tasks and chores, dealing with disagreements and grumpy tired days, are all things that couples who have new babies face together. However, when there is birth trauma in the mix, the challenge becomes much harder. Trauma causes the stress centres of our brain to remain activated even after the danger is over. This is because our mind and body are trying to protect us. The deep-seated part of our brain still feels as though it is in danger. This makes us quick to feel stressed, anxious, panicky, agitated and angry (hallmark symptoms of the 'intrusive' symptoms of PTSD).

Anger is a defence mechanism that has evolved to deal with threat, and it is one which is likely to be triggered against your partner. It can express itself in many ways, and it may seem illogical, as it did in Ruth's case. We met Ruth in Chapters 1 and 3, and her husband, Mike, tells his story in Chapter 5. Whilst she was suffering from PTSD, she would often fly into a rage at her husband for things that would not have seemed important before – for example, maybe he was two minutes late back from shopping. For Ruth this was linked to a desperate need to be in control, which was related to having felt completely out of control during the birth. Or you might feel that your anger is logical. You might feel angry towards your partner because he or she just 'allowed' the birth to take its wrong turn, and didn't protect you or fight for you. In my experience, this is quite common. What is interesting is that when the trauma is resolved, the feeling often shifts. It moves from 'I am so angry at him for not intervening to protect me', to 'I know he was trying his best, and he did try, but the odds were stacked against him too', or 'He was also frightened'. In Ruth's case, during therapy, the anger moved from 'Why can't you just do what I say when I say it?' to 'He really has been through so much, it's a miracle that he stuck by me'. The anger that can come about following birth trauma will, of course, impact on the relationship. Your partner will likely struggle to support you, and may respond to your anger with their own anger. They might feel guilty for their role in what happened. All these can add to the feeling of anger. The negativity between you can escalate, damaging the loving bond and support that you may have had before the birth. The impact that birth trauma can have on your relationship is one really good reason why I would recommend that you get help, because once the trauma is resolved, it is so much easier to navigate the day-to-day strains of living with a new baby, and finding ways to feel connected and support each other through the adventure of parenting.

YOUR RELATIONSHIP WITH YOUR BABY

Birth trauma can affect how quickly we bond with our babies. In a way, this is obvious. If you were traumatised when your baby was born, then it is probable that when you first met him, you were not feeling the love. If your body was still in survival mode, awash with stress hormones, or if you were drugged up or utterly exhausted, the chances are that you felt indifference, or rejection, rather than love. In one study, it was found that all six of the traumatised women researchers spoke to felt rejection towards their babies (Ayers et al, 2007). So you are not alone. Not loving your baby is taboo in our culture, but it needs to be talked about, because medicalisation of childbirth, and maternity wards which are sometimes brutal towards mothers, are adding to the problem. If you were hoping to feel a rush of love when you saw your baby, and you didn't, that is not your fault. By all means be disappointed, and feel the grief of what could have been. But it doesn't make you a bad mother. It does not mean you failed your baby. It does not mean that it can't be fixed. The research has shown that feelings of rejection were temporary. Over time, bonding happens. We put enormous pressure on ourselves as new parents, including the pressure to love our baby fully and instantly. However, this is unrealistic and unfair. If you have had a terrifying labour, then your body wasn't primed to be suddenly calm and loving when the baby was born. You have been through a process in which you were so scared that your brain became flooded with adrenaline and cortisol – those are hormones which are not conducive to love and attachment.

Falling in love with your baby can take a long time, especially if you are in need of emotional healing. All the advice in this book about taking care of yourself so that your healing hormones can be activated will help. This is particularly relevant to falling in love with your baby, because the same hormones are involved for relaxation as they are for love: the calm and connect hormone of oxytocin, and endorphins. Go easy on yourself. Give it time. Take care of yourself as best you can, because that increases the chances of your mind and body being able to fall in love with your baby. Cultures which give the mother and baby time to bond in peace know that at least a month is needed for that to begin to happen. It does not necessarily happen in the first few minutes.

If, after many months, you are finding that you still feel indifferent to your baby, ask yourself 'If someone said I could swap my baby for another baby, would I be okay with that?' The answer is probably no, suggesting that you do have a bond with your baby, but that it is being interrupted by stress. Keep working on the tips and techniques in this book, outlined in Chapters 4 and 8. If, however, the answer is 'yes', then it's time to get some professional help to enable you to bond with your baby by addressing the birth trauma. In some cases, it is not just that mothers are indifferent to their babies, but they can also feel hostile and triggered by their babies. If you are finding that your baby is a trigger to your anxiety, because your brain associates him with the trauma, and as a result you are avoiding him, or interacting with him in a negative way, or having persistent feelings of anger towards him, then it is time to get some help. Remember that this is not your fault, and that trauma is fairly easy to treat. Once you get the PTSD treated, you will have a much better chance of beginning to feel connected to your baby, bonded to him, and able to enjoy his company.

It may be that the birth has done the opposite for you – rather than problems bonding with your baby, you constantly feel frightened and anxious about his welfare. If something happened that was frightening during the birth (or in pregnancy, or after the birth), then this might have left its mark traumatically, and you might find that you become irrationally anxious over any little sign that reminds you of that. For example, Yvonne's baby was rushed into NICU after turning blue in her arms. He was treated, and came back home. However, she couldn't leave him to sleep for fear that he would turn blue again, and she wouldn't notice. She would stay up at night watching him for fear of it happening again. She knew this wasn't logical, but the trauma made it impossible for her to relax and get any rest for herself. Treatment for the trauma made a huge difference. Jessica found that she would always rush to make things better if her daughter was ever upset, because her daughter's distress reignited the guilt that she had felt at the birth. She had always felt that she had let her daughter down at the birth, and the guilt was activated every time her daughter was unhappy. She was aware, on a logical level, that she was treating her two daughters differently, and that it wasn't healthy to rush to her daughter's rescue every time she cried, but her emotional traumatised brain still over-reacted every time. Releasing the trauma helped her to respond to both daughters in a healthier way.

If you feel that your birth trauma has left its mark on your relationship with your baby, then do follow the self-help guides in Chapter 4, and/or seek some form of therapy, as outlined in Chapter 8. They are all designed to help your brain to release the trauma, by producing hormones associated with relaxation, love and calm, rather than with stress and fear. Practising breathing and mindful techniques while you are with your baby is a great bonding exercise. Maybe you can take two minutes out of the day to breathe with your baby, noticing your baby's breathing rhythm and your own. Or you could spend some time while you are holding your baby mindfully noticing five things you can see in your baby, and five things you can feel. Take time to gently look into his eyes, or take time to kiss your baby, noticing how that feels and how your baby responds.

If you have a particularly fussy baby, you might choose to do this while they sleep. Most parents would agree that it is easier to feel loving towards our babies when they are asleep! Don't rush the bonding process. It's never too late, but if you rush it or pressure yourself, then you are in danger of turning it into a stressful venture, rather than the relaxed one that it needs to be.

YOUR SEX LIFE

Your sex life will be altered when a baby arrives, even if you have not been traumatised. Having a new baby in your life is a challenge for any couple's sex life. Add trauma into the mix, and we have even more disruption. Remember that trauma activates our stress centres, which dampen the loving, relaxing parts of our circuitry. If you are suffering from PTSD, then your mind and body will struggle to relax enough to enjoy sexual intimacy. Your brain will struggle with sex just as it struggles with sleep, for the same reason: if you don't feel safe, then you can't switch off and relax. Furthermore, if you are feeling angry towards your partner, as mentioned above, or you don't feel supported or understood, then you are also less likely to want to have sex.

With trauma and PTSD, it may be that your intrusions, flashbacks and triggers can be set off by intimate contact. Maybe being touched in a certain way reminds you of the birth, and causes you to freeze. Maybe the thought of having sex is stressful because the thought of getting pregnant is terrifying. Maybe your partner is having flashbacks of what he or she saw, and when they go to touch you, they are reminded of those images. Maybe the birth served to reignite memories of sexual abuse from way back in your history, but it has all resurfaced now, affecting your current sex life. Whatever your specific stresses might be, if they are being caused or aggravated by upsetting memories of your birth, then that is a sign of trauma, and trauma is relatively easy to treat.

– 8 –

RECOVERING FROM PERINATAL TRAUMA: GETTING PROFESSIONAL HELP

Let me tell you Ruth's story of recovery. It is an example of how getting the correct help can make a monumental difference (we were introduced to Ruth in Chapter 1). Ruth came for therapy four years after her traumatic birth. In that time, she had steadily got worse and worse. Before the birth, she described herself as someone with 'get up and go', someone who looked after herself, had a lot of energy, used to go running and swimming. She was a keen traveller and had built a successful career as a teacher. She described herself as a kind and gentle person. She had looked forward to becoming a mum, having had a healthy and happy pregnancy. However, all that changed after the traumatic birth. When she first came to me, she was a prisoner in her own home. She found it almost impossible to do any more than the bare minimum of taking care of her son. Sometimes she didn't get out of bed. Her garden was untended, her morale was at rock bottom, and she had become inactive, miserable and trapped in a cycle of inertia, rage and guilt. She had cycles of rages, aimed at those nearest to her, and these cycles would leave her feeling ashamed, deeply depressed and suicidal. The depths of her problems culminated in her disappearing one day during a rage, and she was subsequently found walking the wrong way up a dual carriageway, in a disorientated state. She was diagnosed with bipolar depression, and given medication which didn't seem to help. The birth trauma went undiagnosed. I don't tell you this to scare you. I tell you this to let you know that no matter how bad it seems, it can get better.

Within three sessions of trauma-focused therapy, Ruth already felt remarkably different. There were different layers of trauma for Ruth (the horror and distress were one layer, and the rages and need for control were another), and there were some patterns that had been there so long that they took a little while to unravel during therapy. So overall, it took 20 sessions. But after that, she told me she felt normal. That word, 'normal', is a big deal when you aren't well. She was able to talk about the birth, she was running again, helping out at school, managing bad days quickly and effectively, and tending to her garden once again. She was recovered enough to not need any more therapy. She had tried different therapists, and found one that felt right for her. If you know that you would like some professional help, don't hesitate to 'shop around' and find a therapist who specialises in trauma, one that feels right for you.

MAKING THE DECISION TO TAKE THE PLUNGE

Ruth knew she needed help. However, it isn't always that straightforward. Procrastination and finding reasons not to look for professional help are all too common. There are many ways in which you might do this. You might think 'I'm coping okay for now, I'll just crack on with life and make do'. You might think 'I've no idea where to start getting the right help, so I'll leave it for now'. Procrastination is common for one reason: seeking help can be a scary thing to do. We are entering into the unknown. We might share some fears associated with stigma – 'What if people will judge me, what if they think I'm not a good mum, what if they open a can of worms and make me worse?' If you are wrestling with whether or not to seek help, this chapter should help by giving you a better idea of what you might expect when you seek help, and how to seek it. Firstly, let's look at the stages that you will go through in actually seeking professional help.

ARE YOU GOING THROUGH THE STAGES OF CHANGE?

Prochaska and DiClemente put forward a very useful model that you can use to guide you through the process of seeking and finding help. It was originally devised to help us understand how we decide to come off alcohol or drugs, but I think it's also useful to think about it in terms of deciding to seek therapy. The process of change involves all these stages, and you can move backwards and forwards between each stage as you go through the process of getting help for your birth trauma.

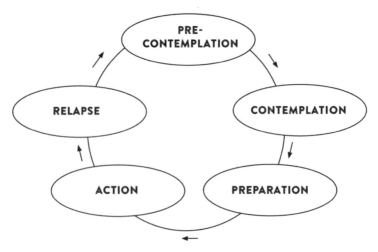

Prochaska and DiClemente, Stages of Change (1983)

Pre-contemplation is the first phase, and it involves having no concept or intention to change at all. This might involve the thought that 'I'm not nearly as bad as Ruth was, so I don't need help'. Or 'Of course I'm upset about the birth, that doesn't mean I need to seek help for it'. Or you might say to your partner when they suggest it 'Why would you think I need help? Do you think I'm losing it or something?'

Contemplation is the second stage. This is where you begin to think about the *possibility* of change. This might involve thinking 'Maybe it could be useful for me,' or 'I might do it one day, but life's too rammed at the moment,' or 'That is something that I do want to do, but no idea when or how'. You can move between contemplation and pre-contemplation on and off for a long time before moving on to stage three.

Preparation is the third stage. You have decided to do something, and you are starting to pull together a plan. You might be asking around, or doing some reading around the options; you may have searched some local therapists, or asked a few friends. You may even have been to the GP and they have given you the number of someone to call. You can move between preparation and contemplation for many months too, in that although you have the number to call, you switch back to 'I'll do it later when I'm less busy' and so on.

Action is the fourth stage. You actually go and talk to a professional about the help that you would like. You have done all the preparation in terms of setting up the appointment, sorting out how to get there, getting in your car or on the bus, and actually turning up. If this goes well, you will find the help that you need to recover from your trauma, and thereby leave the process of making the change. You leave the cycle. If, however, it doesn't go so well, you 'relapse', or rather, change gets paused, and you go back through the cycle once again. You might step back in at pre-contemplation with 'I knew it wasn't right for me, I'm not going to see a professional,' or you might go back to any of the other stages, such as 'preparation', which might involve getting back onto your search engine or going back to your GP, or you might step back in at 'contemplation' knowing that you need to do something, but not quite getting around to doing something about it just yet. Finding the right form of help can involve going around the cycle of change a few times. Don't be discouraged. Keep looking for the right kind of help for you, because it can make such a huge difference to how you feel and to your future.

So, which professionals might help you in your mission to recover from your birth trauma? We will look at what is available in the NHS first, and then move onto other options.

GETTING PROFESSIONAL HELP: THE NHS ROUTE

Services in the NHS are based on recommendations found in the NICE guidelines (NICE stands for National Institute of Clinical Excellence). Basically, professionals in the relevant field get together and review and collate existing evidence relevant to an area of medicine, and then they publish their findings. These are then used as a guide for the NHS to make decisions about which services to pay for and offer. If you are in the UK, NICE guidelines can give you an idea of what the NHS will and will not provide. If you are not in the UK, they can be a useful summary of the research that is out there, especially if you particularly want an approach that is scientifically validated. You can find them online and they are free to access. At the moment, the guidelines suggest that women who are suffering after a traumatic birth (women who have lost babies are included in this) should be offered 'advice and support' if they wish to talk about their experience. They also say that the NHS should 'take into account the effect of the birth or miscarriage on the partner and encourage them to accept support from family and friends'. In terms of treatment, they suggest that women who have PTSD receive one of two interventions. These are trauma-focused CBT or eye-movement desensitisation and reprocessing (EMDR). Let's take a closer look at each of these.

TRAUMA-FOCUSED CBT

Cognitive behavioural therapy is an established form of psychological therapy that has been rigorously 'tested' in randomised controlled trials and been shown to be effective. CBT has been adapted specifically for treating PTSD, and I advise that you ensure that you get a CBT therapist who has gone on to do specific training in CBT for trauma. Treatment involves between six and 18 sessions, during which the goal is to find ways to help you to process the trauma in a way that is tolerable to you. CBT is collaborative, which means that you will be expected to take part in the therapy by doing exercises at home to aid your recovery. You will be focusing on your feelings, your beliefs and your behaviours associated with the trauma, and the therapist will help you to adapt some of these to lift the traumatic symptoms of anxiety, nightmares, avoidance, and so on. The therapist should be sensitive to what feels okay for you, and should help you to feel safe and to go at your own pace. This is important because if you are scared, then the brain will not process the memory as effectively (the amygdala will fire up and thereby block new information from being processed. See Chapter 3 for a review of this theory). It can take a bit of courage to embark on trauma-focused CBT because you will be taking a look at something that basically scares you. But your therapist will help to alleviate any anxiety, and trust me, it's worth it!

EMDR

EMDR stands for Eye Movement Desensitisation and Reprocessing. You may have come across it as 'the one where the therapist holds their two fingers upright, a little way in front of your face, and moves their fingers rapidly from side to side in front of your eyes'. You keep your eyes focused on the moving fingers, while you think of a memory associated with the trauma. It sounds a little odd, but the research is clear: it can help release the symptoms of trauma. Once again, you would be doing a 'course' of EMDR, with treatment ranging from six to 18 sessions. The therapist should go at your pace, and ensure that you feel safe and in control during the process. One of the theories as to why this method works suggests that EMDR mimics a dreaming state (remember that when we dream, our eyes move rapidly, also known as rapid eye movement sleep, or REM sleep). While in a relaxed state, the brain can re-experience the trauma differently and process it, and put it into historic memory. Trauma-focused CBT is doing the same thing, but it may take longer because it doesn't have the automatic benefit of the 'dissociated' and relaxed state that the rapid eye movement will trigger during EMDR. Most areas of England have some form of maternal mental health provision, and you should be able to access those services via your GP, midwife or health visitor. EMDR may be available through the maternal mental health team, or through the general adult mental health team. Either way, don't hesitate to ask for it specifically, as it might not be automatically offered to you.

SPECIALIST PERINATAL MENTAL HEALTH SERVICES

There are a few midwifery services popping up across the country that are trauma-informed and trauma-trained (I know because I've done some of the training). Hopefully, there will be more and more of these, given that the government has put aside money to develop perinatal mental health services across the country. Some of these services offer the rewind method of lifting trauma to women, which is, in my opinion, the most gentle and safest way to work with trauma. However, the NICE guidelines say 'do not offer single-session high-intensity psychological interventions with an explicit focus on "reliving" their trauma to women who have a traumatic birth'. This is because, when done badly, there is a risk of re-traumatisation, and if you are suffering from full-blown PTSD you are going to need to be in experienced hands. However, if you don't meet the criteria for full-blown PTSD and thus can't be referred to a perinatal mental health team, you might want to check out what your midwifery service offers. Some offer valuable, sensitive ways of helping you to come to terms with what happened.

THINGS THE NHS MIGHT OFFER YOU, BUT YOU MIGHT WANT TO DECLINE

Your GP might make some suggestions for you that are generic to mental health, in that they are good for treating depression and anxiety. For example, they may refer you for counselling, they may offer anti-depressants, or they may refer you to IAPT services. IAPT stands for Improvement in Accessing Psychological Therapies. It is a service whereby you will be offered a limited number of CBT sessions, administered by a specifically trained therapist, to target anxiety and depression. It is not guaranteed to be trauma-specific, however, so if you are pretty sure that you are suffering from trauma, it would be worth specifying that you want treatment for trauma, in the form of trauma-focused CBT or EMDR. Similarly, your GP might want to refer you to counselling. However, if you have PTSD, counselling is not always the best course of action, and in some cases, it can make things worse, as getting you to talk about the trauma, without understanding how to lift it, can exacerbate the trauma. As mentioned above, another service that you might be offered is some form of debriefing service with a midwife, during which they will go over your birth notes with you. Again, this can make things worse, because it can dredge up a lot of distress, but not help you to process or relieve the actual trauma.

To summarise, it may seem that there isn't much out there for you, but if you persist, and talk to your midwife, your GP and your health visitor, you should, in the end, find that you can get help via the NHS. Good luck!

GETTING PROFESSIONAL HELP: THE PRIVATE ROUTE

There are many options out there for private therapy routes. These might include psychologists, counsellors, psychotherapists, hypnotherapists, hypnobirthing instructors, Emotional Freedom practitioners (EFT), breath-work therapists and osteopaths, along with a host of energy therapies that aim to release distress and trauma in their own special way. I work with many wonderful therapists who are doing some incredible work to alleviate the enormous distress that is out there among women who are upset about their births. They are not recognised by the NHS, or by NICE guidelines, and their valuable work can often be minimised or disregarded or even held in disdain by the dominant patriarchy, which prefers to hail anything explained by science as the holy grail in healing, over and above the lived experience of millions of people. Pharmaceutical intervention is the most highly regarded, and stays dominant.

Energy healers, who do not (yet) have the power of science behind them, remain at the bottom of the heap, belittled and scoffed at by those who hold the power. It is not a new pattern. Five hundred years ago, traditional healers and midwives, who used herbs and wisdom passed down through generations, were forcibly replaced by medical doctors (being a midwife was outlawed unless you had been trained, and training was banned for women). Midwives were viewed as dangerous and ignorant, and are still being accused of those things today. In contrast, doctors were held in high esteem, and given more status, power and money, despite causing deaths in their droves through childbed fever caused by their poor hand hygiene. Even today, if a woman dies at the hands of a doctor, the doctor is not scrutinised in the same way that a midwife is.

A doctor is paid so much more. A doctor's worth is seen and respected more than that of a midwife. Compassionate care saves lives, but it is not valued in the same way. Healthcare is a feminist issue, and delivering healthcare is a social power tool. I am speaking as a member of a valued profession: clinical psychology has managed to stay well paid, well respected and valued in this culture. Perhaps this is because men are well represented in the profession, making up around 30% of practitioners, although this is declining, as is the standard rate of payment. As a clinical psychologist, I want to give a shout out to some of the effective and valuable therapists that are out there, which you can access via the internet and by word-of-mouth recommendations.

There are, of course, some cowboys out there, as there are in any profession, both inside the NHS and outside it. By all means, do your research. You might want to make sure of any practitioner's professional training, and that they continue to be registered by a professional or governing body. This means that there is a little more reassurance that they abide by ethical and professional boundaries, that they continue to do what is required of them by their profession, such as ongoing training, or ongoing mentoring and supervision, and that any complaints from the public have been responded to. Some examples of relevant governing bodies include the Health and Care Professions Council (HCPC), the British Psychological Society (BPS), the British Association of Behavioural and Cognitive Psychotherapies (BABCP), and the EMDR Association. It is possible for one therapist to be a member of all of these associations at once. It is also possible for a counsellor to be registered with the British Association of Counselling, but to have no training or experience in treatment of trauma, so do check their specialisms as well as their professional qualifications.

In the previous section of this chapter, we looked at trauma-based CBT and EMDR as viable therapy options for lifting trauma. These therapies can be administered by a range of therapy professionals, such as clinical psychologists, CBT therapists, psychotherapists and more. Within the private sector, there are two therapy approaches that we will now look at. As before, these can be administered by a range of private therapists, such as counsellors, psychotherapists, clinical psychologists, hypnotherapists and more. They are the tool to do the therapy with. These therapies are not easy to access in the NHS, but I think that they are valuable options for lifting symptoms of trauma following birth.

EMOTIONAL FREEDOM TECHNIQUE (EFT)

This method of treating birth trauma was mentioned in the chapter on self-help. It is not recommended in the NICE guidelines – yet. But it is exciting that this gentle and effective technique has sparked enough interest from NICE for it to recommend that money be invested in further research. So far, the evidence suggests that it works, but NICE suggests that it needs a bit more rigorous scientific testing to be able to be absolutely clear about its benefits.

I am not an EFT therapist, so Tricia Murray, an expert in the field, has kindly offered to tell us about it in her own words. Tricia specialises in working therapeutically with families in the perinatal period.

EFT (also known as 'Tapping') is becoming recognised as an effective intervention for PTSD. It was recently included in the NICE (2018) guidelines for PTSD, recognising that there was enough evidence specifically for PTSD to be worthy of government-funded further research. Studies have found EFT results in changes in the brain, DNA expression, hormone production, brain waves, and blood flow. It is also recognised as being relatively quick with no adverse effects. It works like other talking therapies and at the same time stimulates various points on the hands, head, face and body through tapping. These points regulate the nervous system and elicit a sense of calm in the body. Through this process, the person feels calm when they bring to mind the issue. What's brilliant about EFT is we can work directly with how the body is responding. We don't need words or explanations. Often women leave my sessions, even if it's been really challenging, telling me how relaxed they feel, as though they've had a massage, yet it's only their own fingers that have tapped on their body. Once someone has learned how to use it, they can also support themselves between sessions (for example, if they experience a flashback or panic attack) or to keep supporting themselves after the therapy sessions are complete. It is suited to PTSD/trauma symptoms because it's gentle, it works with the physical symptoms in the body as well as the mind, it's relatively quick, it's easy for people to learn and if they choose to integrate it into their lives, they can. Typically, it might take four to eight sessions to support recovery from a traumatic event such as birth trauma.

If you want to give this a go, Tricia recommends the EFT International (eftinternational.org) as a place to start looking for someone to suit you. Their accredited practitioners undergo a rigorous accreditation process, and adhere to ongoing membership criteria regarding ethics, supervisory codes and continuing professional development.

THE REWIND METHOD FOR LIFTING TRAUMA

The rewind method for lifting trauma, a term originally coined by David Muss, has been adapted by the Human Givens Institute from a long-standing hypnotherapy technique known as the 'visual/kinaesthetic dissociation technique'. It is gaining popularity among midwives working with birth trauma, because it is a gentle, effective way to relieve symptoms of trauma. I have been using the rewind method with my clients for many years with dramatic results. I rarely do trauma-focused CBT anymore, because I find it more distressing for the client, and it takes longer, and isn't as effective in my experience. I have been training midwives in the method too. It is suitable for people who are distressed after a birth, and struggling to move on, but who do *not* meet the criteria for full-blown PTSD (when they can be referred to mental health services). Unfortunately, NICE do not recommend it at the current time. This might be due to concern about the fact that the rewind method is a tool which isn't regulated in the same way as CBT or EMDR. As with any psychological therapy tool, if misunderstood or misused it could re-traumatise the client. Having said that, this applies to counselling and debriefing services too, which have both been known to make things worse, and yet debriefing services are not regulated or audited in the NHS. In the words of the Human Givens Institute:

Extensive clinical experience shows it to be a more cost-effective and successful treatment than the treatments recommended by NICE guidelines, namely CBT and EMDR, that take many sessions and are often only partially successful. Treatment is safe (unlike critical incident debriefing for example, which research shows may increase rates of PTSD). Treatment is non-voyeuristic (it is suitable for victims of sexual assault, beating or any kind of humiliation, as the victim do not have to tell the therapist details what happened.) Treatment is fast.

All of the case studies in this book were from clients of mine who benefitted from the rewind method in their therapy with me. Some recovered in two sessions. One recovered after less than 20 sessions, having suffered four years of suicidality, dangerous behaviours and a diagnosis of bipolar disorder – a diagnosis which turned out to be erroneous. It was PTSD, and all she needed was some focused trauma therapy. I am a huge advocate of this method, and one of the things I love most about it is that it can be used by people in the caring professions who aren't highly trained psychotherapists. You can even do it yourself! If you have been traumatised by your birth, but you do not meet the diagnostic criteria for a mental health disorder such as PTSD, and you can find a practitioner who is a member of a professional body, and who is trained in the rewind method, and who comes recommended, then I would say give it a go. It might just change your life.

ALTERNATIVE THERAPIES

There are plenty of alternative therapies which purport to help ease the symptoms of trauma. They include yoga, massage, reiki, breath work, acupuncture and aromatherapy. At the very least, these might help you to feel better and strengthen you a little to help you cope with a very challenging time in your life. However, I suspect that they do way more than that. We know enough to be able to say that these therapies will help activate your relaxation/calm response, thereby potentially assisting your nervous system to kick-start the neurological changes necessary to shift the traumatic memory from the amygdala to the neocortex. They might activate your placebo effect, giving you a valuable, safe and healthy means of recovery. They might also do things which science can't yet measure or explain. If you feel that a therapy will help you, then I would suggest you try it. The same guidelines apply – find a therapist who is a member of some kind of governing body, so that they are regulated and accountable.

– 9 –

THE NEXT PREGNANCY AND BEYOND

CONSIDERING ANOTHER BABY

If you have had a previous traumatic birth, it is completely normal to feel scared when you think about getting pregnant again. When you think about the prospect, there may be a sense of dread. Other people might be telling you that it'll be fine, and it won't be the same, and other reassuring things like that. But deep down, you are still frightened. Or maybe there is no way you are going to entertain the thought of another pregnancy because the fear is too strong. You can't contemplate doing it again, and so you are resigning yourself to never having another baby. Or maybe you ignore the issue, letting the years slip by until it becomes apparent that it won't ever happen. Alternatively, you might make an active decision not to have another child. If you choose to avoid having another baby because of the trauma, I want you to come to that decision with peace and with acceptance. I don't want you to be left feeling regret, or guilty, and I don't want you to be left feeling bitter and angry.

One of the problems with deciding not to have another baby based on a previous traumatic birth is when it is a decision based on avoidance and fear alone. It is restricting you: the fear is the motivator. The decision not to have another baby as a result of a previous traumatic birth is a decision that I would fully support, as long as that decision has not been made in fear *alone*, and has been worked through. You might choose to take a look at the stages of grief outlined in Chapter 6, so that you come to a place of acceptance and peace, knowing that it is the right thing for you and your family to not try for any more babies. This will free you up to go on and enjoy the rest of your life without 'what ifs' or 'why didn't I's' or 'I should haves'. Presuming there is a co-parent involved, it also means talking it through with them, and jointly grieving/processing/ being okay with the decision. This is something you might choose to do with a counsellor, or with your partner, or with a very good friend.

WHEN YOU DO WANT ANOTHER BABY BUT YOU ARE SCARED

However, because you are reading this section of the book, you might be in the same boat as a lot of other women who have had traumatic births. You might want another baby deep down, but you are really very scared to do so. You want a baby, but you can't contemplate having a baby. You are stuck. This kind of fear can become so strong that it leaves you very miserable, or it can affect your daily life. For example, you might feel so frightened that you avoid sex, despite having a number of contraceptives in place, because the fear of getting pregnant again is too great. You are not alone. I can guarantee that you are not alone, not just because I have heard it directly from the mouths of hundreds of women, but also because there is even a name for this dread. It is known as secondary tokophobia. Tokophobia is a fear of childbirth, and secondary means that it concerns the second (or more) baby, and has been caused directly as a result of witnessing or experiencing a previous traumatic birth. In order to overcome tokophobia, you need to treat the trauma. This is the role of a trauma specialist, as outlined in Chapter 8. Treatment for secondary tokophobia is not just about trauma release: there will be other aspects of the treatment which are necessary, such as helping you to consider a future pregnancy. Once you have had treatment for tokophobia, you might still feel apprehensive, but hopefully, you will feel well enough to consider another pregnancy.

PREPARING FOR ANOTHER BABY FOLLOWING A TRAUMATIC BIRTH

So, what can you do? When I was a hypnobirthing practitioner and birth doula, my job was often to help a mum overcome her previous traumatic birth and help her towards a healing subsequent birth. It is very possible. Preparation is key. I know that you can't control the outcome of your birth, but you can certainly put things in place to increase the likelihood of things going well for you.

1 **If you haven't already, de-traumatise yourself from the first birth.** Use the tips and techniques in this book to help yourself to recover. If the phobia is bad, or you do not feel like you have recovered despite putting into place the things suggested in this book, find a therapist to help you. That is what they are there for. If you had a bad back, and despite doing exercises to fix it, it still hurt, you would go to a specialist. It's the same with your brain and nervous system. Doulas can be especially useful because they have a good grasp of how the maternity system can traumatise us, and they work all the time with women who are frightened of birth for various reasons. My advice would be to find one with training and experience in trauma.

2 **Gather your team.** The second step is to take control of your birth by enlisting the help of people who can help you have a voice. It might take a bit of detective work to do this part.

You might look to the private sector, such as a birth doula, or an independent midwife. It might involve people in the NHS, such as consultant midwives, or a midwife in the community who you know and trust, or the head of the maternity ward, or a consultant obstetrician who comes recommended and who really listens to you. Sometimes a local doula can help you to link up with the right professionals. The NHS is equipped to work with women who have needs beyond the usual; it's just a matter of knowing how to access that. Once you have found a professional who you feel respects you and listens to you, I suggest that you tell them about your traumatic birth. If you have a history of trauma previous to that, especially a history of sexual assault or abuse, then if you feel able to, it can also help to let them know about that. They should tailor your care accordingly, for example, writing a tailored birth plan with you, and maybe even providing some continuity of care, depending on your local maternity service. Research suggests that having a supportive midwifery team is even more important if there has been previous trauma. They will help you to think about what kind of birth you would like this time around. For example, you might know that you want an elective caesarean section this time. Or you might know that you want a home birth. Or you might know that you want an epidural as early as possible. You will be surprised how much choice you legally have when it comes to childbirth. You might have been told 'you aren't allowed' or 'you have to', but this simply isn't true. In the UK, it is your body, your birth, and if you want to do something that goes against medical advice, that is your right. Finding professionals to support you is the key. If they are up-to-date in their training, they will also be aware of your rights and will support you in them.

3 **Prepare your mind.** Once you start to get a team behind you, and feel more optimistic because of that, you might find that you feel better. However, every now and again the old anxiety or dread might creep back in. This is normal, but it can be alleviated by remembering to take care of yourself by activating your relaxation/oxytocin system. Remember that your relaxation system is the antidote to your stress system. There are many great ways of doing this out there at the moment. I would recommend Mindful Mamma's programmes (I am biased in this. I co-wrote the package with Sophie Fletcher and taught it for many years. There are other hypnobirthing options out there too!). You can download audio relaxation MP3s, or, even better, take one of the one-day classes designed to help you release fear at a subconscious level (from the amygdala).

4 **Don't be frightened to write a birth plan.** Maybe the term 'birth preferences' works better, because you can't control how your birth will pan out, but you can communicate the things that matter to you to the staff who will be serving you. Your preferences will probably be influenced by what you found traumatic last time. For example, you might want to put 'Please communicate what is happening to me throughout, especially in the event of an emergency'. Or you might put 'I was traumatised from my last birth, and as a result I am anxious about this birth', or 'Please note that I might not be able to communicate when I am getting very anxious, but my partner will know, and they will tell you', and so forth. When writing your birth preferences, it is best to work through them with the help of your support team. Also, ask them how they will communicate your needs, for when you go into labour. The next birth is often a chance to be clearer about your wishes and needs, no matter how different they may seem. For example, you might not actually, deep down, want your partner to be at the birth with you. It might be that he doesn't want to be there either, especially if he has secondary tokophobia from a previous birth, or was traumatised in some way. This is your chance to think about what you actually want, and find a way to communicate those needs and preferences. Write them down in a birth plan, and talk them through with your care providers.

5 If you have the funds, I would always recommend hiring a birth doula. She will help you to prepare for the birth and she will be able to provide valuable information about local services. She does not replace your birth partner. Far from it: she supports him or her too. During the birth, she will do whatever you want her to do. Sometimes, the doula is just a 'safety net' and stays in the background while you labour, and while your partner provides all the loving support you need. Sometimes the doula just watches carefully, making sure you are okay from a distance, and only steps in if you seem to be getting upset or something needs doing. She can be your voice, ensuring that the staff are aware of your needs, and helping you to feel supported in the event that anything does feel frightening or out of control for you.

6 Write a postnatal care plan. This is something that is gaining popularity, but I'd like to see it integrated into everyone's birth preparation, because I think it is so useful for mental wellbeing generally. In fact, in my eyes, it is so important, that I have given it its own subheading. Read on to find out why and how to create your own postnatal care plan.

HOW TO WRITE YOUR OWN POSTNATAL CARE PLAN

Many other cultures, both across the globe and going back in time, take care of their new mothers. For the first 6 weeks after birth, mothers are expected to rest in bed and do very little other than be with their baby. Our society isn't so good at that. On the contrary, there tends to be an emphasis on 'getting back to normal' as soon as possible. getting back home, getting back into their jeans, getting up and about and exercising and cleaning. If our society isn't going to take care of you, and if you don't have a 'village' to feed you and nurture you as they do in other cultures, then you're going to have to do it yourself. The idea is that you plan the days after you've had your baby carefully, aiming to maximise your healing and your bonding with your baby. This used to be known as the babymoon period – the time when you get to know your baby physically, and fall in love with them (a honeymoon was for the same purpose of getting to know your new spouse and cementing that relationship physically). Put aside a good budget for this – it's more important than the cot and travel system, because it is about you, your baby and your future together. There are two aims generally. Firstly, freeing up time so that the three of you can bond and rest. How do you do this? Delegate as much as possible! Housework, cooking, shopping, cleaning, bed-changing, washing, and so on. Plan who is going to do it and when. Pay for it, call in favours, or postpone it. The second goal of a postnatal care plan is to make sure that you incorporate lots of quality time for recovery and bonding. Remember that the bonding hormone which mediates bonding and recovery is oxytocin, so we want oxytocin-rich activities, such as relaxation, meditation, massage, snoozing in bed, watching smoochy films, eating chocolate (well, that's actually associated with endorphins, but endorphins are relaxation hormones too, so if you like chocolate, go for it), deep bubbly baths, lots of cuddles, aromatherapy, lovely music, and more. The list will be special to you, and of course, because you have a little baby in your life, you will need support from others to see this through, and most activities will need to be instantly interruptible. That is why it is important to get partners involved in this, so they can run the bath, or put the music on, or whatever is in the postnatal care plan. When you write your postnatal care plan, it can help to put in some time frames: for example, what you will do in the first few days, and what you would like in the first week, and then three weeks, and six weeks. For example, you might decide that you're going to stay in bed for three days, stay in your pyjamas for seven days, and stay in the house for fourteen days. There is an example of a postnatal care plan for you in the appendices of this book, which you can use as an outline for creating your own. Have some indulgent fun thinking up all the lovely things you can do. If you end up with a traumatic birth, then it will help you recover more quickly and more easily. However, the chances are that your birth will be just fine, in which case, your babymoon period will be one that you remember for the right reasons, and treasure for the rest of your life.

CONCLUSION

I'm not a poet, but if I were, I would write something about my love of birth, babies, and women. Our society has, for at least 500 years, failed to see the beauty of women's birthing bodies. I would never have thought, in my wildest dreams, that I would be a birth doula. In my naivety, I regarded birth as painful and messy and yucky. I remember my horror when someone asked me whether I could be at her birth. I asked myself, why does that horrify me? Then, in my usual stubborn way, I decided to do doula training, simply to challenge myself. I got hooked somehow. And having attended many births since then, I can tell you that I am now witness to the fact that birth can be powerful, incredible, and a force of nature. Literally a force of nature. I feel, smell, and hear the force of energy, while a woman works to bring her baby earthside. It really is true that a woman's face becomes beautiful as she labours. I guess it's just the effects of the oxytocin. To see that power and force and beauty be brutally damaged and irrevocably smashed by a patriarchal system which knows not what it does, breaks my heart. And that is why I wrote this book. If you have been broken by birth, I am so sorry that this has happened to you. I sincerely hope this book has helped put some of the pieces back together again so that you can feel resilient and powerful; strengthened by what you've had to endure. My respect goes out to you.

REFERENCES

CHAPTER 1

Hera Cook (2005) *The Long Sexual Revolution; English Women, Sex and Contraception 1800–1975*, Oxford University Press.

Susan Ayers, (2014) 'Fear of Childbirth, postnatal post-traumatic stress disorder and midwifery care', Editorial, *Midwifery Journal*, Vol 30, issue 2.

Creedy, D.K., Gamble, J. (2016) 'A third of midwives who have experienced traumatic perinatal events have symptoms of post-traumatic stress disorder', *Evidence-Based Nursing* 19 (44).

Jenny Patterson, (2019) 'Traumatised Midwives; Traumatised Women' *AIMS Journal, Vol 30, No 4.*

CHAPTER 2

Kerstin Uvnas-Moberg (2011) *The Oxytocin Factor: Tapping the Hormone of Calm, Love and Healing,* Pinter & Martin.

Paul Gilbert (2010) *The Compassionate Mind,* Constable and Robinson.

Singer & Klimecki (2014) 'Empathy and compassion', *Current Biology Volume 24, Issue 18.*

Susan Ayers, (2014) 'Fear of Childbirth, postnatal post-traumatic stress disorder and midwifery care', Editorial, *Midwifery Journal*, Vol 30, issue 2.

Shanafelt, T.D. (2009) 'Enhancing the Meaning of Work: A Prescription for Preventing Physician Burnout and Promoting Patient-Centered Care.' *Journal of the American Medical Association*, 302, 2009:1338-1340.

Daniels, Arden-Close and Mayers (2020) 'Be quiet and man up: a qualitative questionnaire study into fathers who witnessed their partner's birth trauma', *BMC Pregnancy and Childbirth* 20:236.

Menage, Bailey, Lees, and Coad, (2020) 'Women's lived experience of compassionate midwifery': *Human and professional Midwifery*

Fukuzawa, Cuthbert (2017) 'Continuous support for women during childbirth'. *Cochrane Database of Systematic Reviews* 2017, Issue 7.

Bernard Lown, MD, (1996) *The Lost Art of Healing: Practicing Compassion in Medicine*. New York: Ballantine Books.

Robin Youngson (2012) *Time to Care; How to Love Your Patients and Your Job,* Rebel Heart.

CHAPTER 3

Kerstin Uvnäs-Moberg (2010) *The Oxytocin Factor; Tapping the Hormone of Calm, Love and Healing* Pinter & Martin.

Ayers, Bond, Bertullies, & Wijma (2016). 'The aetiology of post-traumatic stress following childbirth: A meta-analysis and theoretical framework'. *Psychological Medicine, 46*(06), 1121–1134.

Susan Ayers (2017) editorial, *Journal of Reproductive and Infant Psychology*, Vol 35 (5).

Bohren, Hofmeyr, Sakala, Fukuzawa, & Cuthbert (2017) 'Continuous support for women during childbirth'. Cochrane Database of Systematic Reviews.

Sandall, Soltani, Gates, Shennan, Devane (2016) 'Midwife-led continuity models versus other models of care for childbearing women'. Cochrane database of systematic reviews.

Harris, Ayers (2012) 'What makes labour and birth traumatic? A survey of intrapartum 'hotspots'' *Psychological Health* 27(10):1166-77.

Hollander, van Hastenberg, van Dillen, van Pampus, de Miranda, and Stramrood (2017) 'Preventing traumatic childbirth experiences: 2,192 women's perceptions and views' Arch Womens Mental Health. 20(4): 515–523.

CHAPTER 4

Dikmen-Yildiz, Ayers, Phillips (2017) 'Longitudinal trajectories of post-traumatic stress disorder (PTSD) after birth and associated risk factors'. *Journal of Affective disorders*, Mar 15;229:377-385.

Ayers, Eagle, & Waring (2006) 'The effects of childbirth-related post-traumatic stress disorder on women and their relationships: A qualitative study' *Psychology Health and Medicine* Nov;11(4):389-98.

CHAPTER 6

Gabrielle Palmer (2009) *The Politics of Breastfeeding: When Breasts are Bad for Business* Pinter & Martin.

Amy Brown (2019) *Why Breastfeeding Grief and Trauma Matter* Pinter & Martin.

Daniels, Arden-Close & Mayers (2020) 'Be quiet and man up: a qualitative questionnaire study into fathers who witnessed their Partner's birth trauma' *BMC Pregnancy and Childbirth* Volume 20, Article number: 236.

Patterson, J (2019) 'Traumatised Midwives; Traumatised Women' *AIMS Journal, 2019, Vol 30, No 4.*

Sheen, Spiby & Slade (2015) 'Exposure to traumatic perinatal experiences and post-traumatic stress symptoms in midwives: prevalence and association with burnout' *International Journal of Nursing Studies, 52 (2) 578-87*

APPENDIX 1

Diagnostic and Statistical Manual of Mental Disorders criteria for a diagnosis of Post-Traumatic Stress Disorder

Categories A–H
Criterion A: stressor (one required)
The person was exposed to: death, threatened death, actual or threatened serious injury, or actual or threatened sexual violence, in the following way(s):

- Direct exposure
- Witnessing the trauma
- Learning that a relative or close friend was exposed to a trauma
- Indirect exposure to aversive details of the trauma, usually in the course of professional duties (e.g., first responders, medics)

Criterion B: intrusion symptoms (one required)
The traumatic event is persistently re-experienced in the following way(s):

- Unwanted upsetting memories
- Nightmares
- Flashbacks
- Emotional distress after exposure to traumatic reminders
- Physical reactivity after exposure to traumatic reminders

Criterion C: avoidance (one required)
Avoidance of trauma-related stimuli after the trauma, in the following way(s):

- Trauma-related thoughts or feelings
- Trauma-related external reminders

Criterion D: negative alterations in cognitions and mood (two required)

Negative thoughts or feelings that began or worsened after the trauma, in the following way(s):

- Inability to recall key features of the trauma
- Overly negative thoughts and assumptions about oneself or the world
- Exaggerated blame of self or others for causing the trauma
- Negative affect
- Decreased interest in activities
- Feeling isolated
- Difficulty experiencing positive affect

Criterion E: alterations in arousal and reactivity

Trauma-related arousal and reactivity that began or worsened after the trauma, in the following way(s):

- Irritability or aggression
- Risky or destructive behavior
- Hypervigilance
- Heightened startle reaction
- Difficulty concentrating
- Difficulty sleeping

Criterion F: duration (required)

Symptoms last for more than 1 month.

Criterion G: functional significance (required)

Symptoms create distress or functional impairment (e.g., social, occupational).

Criterion H: exclusion (required)

Symptoms are not due to medication, substance use, or other illness.

APPENDIX 2

EXAMPLE POSTNATAL CARE PLAN

Here is a fictitious example of how a postnatal care plan might look. Use it for some inspiration when writing your own.

I have written a postnatal care plan because I had a traumatic birth last time, and I want to ensure that I get as much recovery as possible this time, by prioritising my physical and mental health. I am aware that I have a tendency to do too much, and to feel guilty when I'm not getting stuff done. I want to ensure that this doesn't happen following the birth of my baby, and so I am planning how to take care of myself in the first two precious weeks with my baby.

Generally, I wish to spend time skin-to-skin with my baby, I wish to establish breastfeeding, and I would like my partner/ mum to be an integral part of this with us.

Immediately upon coming home

- *My partner would like to carry me and our baby over the threshold.*

- *I would like a warm bath with rejuvenating bath salts, and then I would like to get into fresh (new) pyjamas and into our (newly bought) king-size bed with new fresh sheets, and my baby.*

- *I would like the lights kept low, my phone and my remote control next to me.*

- *I would like to eat a huge, warm, filling meal of cottage pie and peas, washed down with camomile tea and a glass of fizz.*

- *I would like my partner to join us as much as possible in bed.*

For the first two weeks after coming home

- *I would like visitors to stay away for at least 12 hours, apart from the midwife and my lactation consultant, who I have pre-arranged support with.*

- *In the first three days, I would like very close members of my family only, to visit.*

- *I do not want my baby to be held by anybody else in the first three days, other than her father.*

- *We have arranged for a food delivery of fresh fruit, salads, sandwiches, chocolates and wine. There are plenty of ready cooked meals in the freezer too.*

- *I have arranged for a cleaner to come in every other day to tidy and clean the house, as per my partner's requests (she will not clean our bedroom).*

- *I have specific herbal/homeopathic remedies that I will be taking each day.*

- *After the first three days, I have arranged for a postnatal doula to come in and provide emotional and practical support every three days.*

- *My partner will help to ensure that I get plenty of rest, by regularly encouraging me to go to bed, and ensuring that the household and visitors are taken care of.*

- *My partner will take a few hours out of the house each day, to do something to help him to feel refreshed too.*

- *According to how I feel, I plan to spend most of the first two weeks in and out of bed. I might take a walk or potter around the house if I feel restless, but if not, I will stay in bed to recover and adjust, both physically and mentally, and to help me to fall in love with my baby and establish breastfeeding.*

- *Thank you so much for helping us to make the first few weeks of our baby's life special and memorable for the right reasons, and for helping me to get the very best start possible on the journey to becoming a mother.*

What do you think? If you are thinking 'that's a bit overindulgent' then remember that this is a very special time in your life, which you will never have again. Be as indulgent as you like! If you are thinking it's only relevant to 'rich people' then drop the champagne and the au pair, but stick with bed and help from family. If you're thinking 'What if I'm a single mum?' then think even harder about your postnatal care plan, because support matters, whether it's from a husband, a mother, the NHS, a best friend or voluntary organisations.

ACKNOWLEDGEMENTS

I don't specifically remember deciding to write this book. I guess I must have talked about the gap in the market, because I do remember Mark Harris encouraging me to go ahead and ask Pinter & Martin if they would support me with it. Without him, I don't think this book would have happened, and for that, I thank him.

I would also like to thank all the women that I have been a psychologist to – women who have allowed me in to their private lives, and shared their gut-wrenching stories of birth trauma. Thank you for that privilege. I sincerely hope that I learnt well from you, and that this book reflects some of all that I have learnt from you over the years. Thank you in particular to those women (and one man) who generously shared their stories in this book. It is very alien to me to ask people to break their confidentiality, and for that reason, asking you all was not easy. But you made it easy by being so generous with your offers of help. I would love to be able to thank my very first birth trauma client over twenty years ago, who sparked my interest in this whole subject. I wish I'd known then, what I know now, for your sake.

Thank you to my husband, who holds the fort while I write, who encourages me when I insist that this writing lark was a stupid idea, and who is always there, steady and steadfast in his support of everything that I do. I would not even have gone into the birthing world in the first place without his encouragement. Thank you from the bottom of my heart, Scott.

Thank you to Martin Wagner, and the Pinter & Martin team who beaver away in the background, somehow magically making this book happen. It's so lovely to have a team behind me – something that I have not experienced in many years. In particular, thank you to Susan Last for starting me on the writing journey in the first place by originally asking me to contribute to the *Why It Matters* series.

And thank you to my incredible circle of friends who bolster me, fulfil me, and refuel me. I guess you get more of a mention at the moment because we are temporarily separated by Covid-19. You know who you are, and you know that I love you.

INDEX

Also from Pinter & Martin

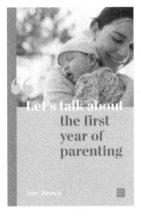

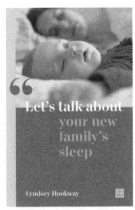

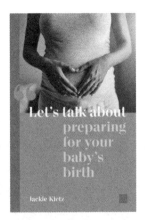

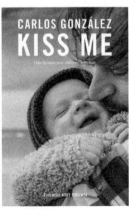

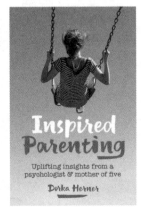

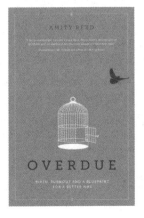

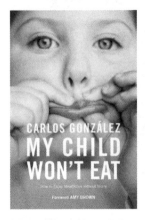

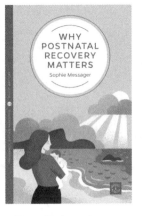

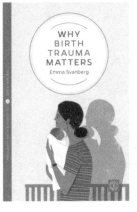

pinterandmartin.com